Problem-Based Learning in Health and Social Care

Problem-Based Learning in Health and Social Care

Edited by

Teena J. Clouston
Lyn Westcott
Steven W. Whitcombe
Jill Riley
Ruth Matheson

WILEY-BLACKWELL

A John Wiley & Sons, Ltd., Publication

This edition first published 2010
© 2010 Blackwell Publishing Ltd

Blackwell Publishing was acquired by John Wiley & Sons in February 2007. Blackwell's publishing programme has been merged with Wiley's global Scientific, Technical, and Medical business to form Wiley-Blackwell.

Registered office
John Wiley & Sons Ltd, The Atrium, Southern Gate, Chichester, West Sussex, PO19 8SQ, United Kingdom

Editorial offices
9600 Garsington Road, Oxford, OX4 2DQ, United Kingdom
350 Main Street, Malden, MA 02148-5020, USA

For details of our global editorial offices, for customer services and for information about how to apply for permission to reuse the copyright material in this book please see our website at www.wiley.com/wiley-blackwell.

Wiley also publishes its books in a variety of electronic formats. Some content that appears in print may not be available in electronic books.

Designations used by companies to distinguish their products are often claimed as trademarks. All brand names and product names used in this book are trade names, service marks, trademarks or registered trademarks of their respective owners. The publisher is not associated with any product or vendor mentioned in this book. This publication is designed to provide accurate and authoritative information in regard to the subject matter covered. It is sold on the understanding that the publisher is not engaged in rendering professional services. If professional advice or other expert assistance is required, the services of a competent professional should be sought.

Library of Congress Cataloging-in-Publication Data

Problem-based learning in health and social care / edited by Teena J. Clouston . . . [et al.].
   p. ; cm.
  Includes bibliographical references and index.
  ISBN 978-1-4051-8056-6 (pbk. : alk. paper) 1. Medicine – Study and teaching. 2. Social work education. 3. Problem-based learning. I. Clouston, Teena J.
  [DNLM: 1. Health Personnel – education. 2. Problem-Based Learning. 3. Social Work – education. W 18 P961905 2010]
  R834.5.P757 2010
  610.76 – dc22

                                                                                    2009049786

A catalogue record for this book is available from the British Library.

Set in 10/12.5 pt Palatino by Laserwords Private Limited, Chennai, India
Printed and bound in Malaysia by Vivar Printing Sdn Bhd

1   2010

Contents

List of Contributors

Dr Gail Boniface, DipCOT, Cert Ed, Cert in Supervisory Management, MEd, PhD
Senior Lecturer/Programme Lead, School of Healthcare Studies, Cardiff University

Teena J. Clouston, MBA, PgDip, SSRM, DipCOT, DipCouns, DipAT, Certhyp, FHEA
Senior Lecturer/Programme Lead, School of Healthcare Studies, Cardiff University

Juan Delport, Consultant Clinical Psychologist, MA, MEd, DClinPsych
Cwm Taf Local Health Board

Susan Delport, BSc (Hons) OT, MSc OT
Lecturer, School of Healthcare Studies, Cardiff University

Liz Galle, BSc (Hons) OT, BSc, RM, RN
Senior Occupational Therapist, Aneurin Bevan LHB, Talygarn Mental Health Unit, County Hospital

Bernhard Haas, MSc, BA (Hons), MCSP, FHEA
Deputy Head of School of Health Professions, University of Plymouth

Andrew Machon, PhD, MA
Executive Consultant

Sandra Marshman, BSc (Hons) OT
Senior Occupational Therapist, Prince Charles Hospital, OT Department, Gurnos Estate, Merthyr Tydfil

Ruth Matheson, MSc, DipCOT, CMS, FHEA
Senior Lecturer, Learning and Teaching Development Unit, University of Wales Institute, Cardiff (UWIC)

Gareth Morgan, BA (Hons), CQSW, PGCE
Lecturer, School of Healthcare Studies, Cardiff University

Sue Pengelly, DipCOT, BA, MBA, FHEA
Lecturer, School of Healthcare Studies, Cardiff University

Dr Jill Riley, PhD, MSc, DipCOT
Lecturer, School of Healthcare Studies, Cardiff University

Gwilym Wyn Roberts, MA, PGDip (Psych), DipCOT
Director of Occupational Therapy, School of Healthcare Studies, Cardiff University

Sara Roberts, MEd, DipCOT
Course Director, School of Healthcare Sciences, Bangor University

Sally Scott-Roberts, DipCOT, MEd
Senior Lecturer – Inclusion, School of Education, University of Wales, Newport

Alison Seymour, MSc, PCUTL, PGCM, BSc, DipCOT
Lecturer, School of Healthcare Studies, Cardiff University

Ruth Squire, DipCOT
Lecturer, School of Healthcare Studies, Cardiff University

Pam Stead, MEd, DipCOT
Lecturer, School of Healthcare Studies, Cardiff University

Lyn Westcott, MSc, BSc, DipCOT, FHEA
Senior Lecturer/Professional Lead – Occupational Therapy, Faculty of Health,
University of Plymouth

Steven W. Whitcombe, MSc, BA (Hons), BSc (Hons) OT, PGCE (PCET), FHEA
Lecturer, School of Healthcare Studies, Cardiff University

1: Starting out: a guide to using this book and its development

Lyn Westcott

When you set out on your journey to Ithaca,
pray that the road is long,
full of adventure, full of knowledge. . . .
Always keep Ithaca on your mind.
To arrive there is your ultimate goal.
But do not hurry the voyage at all.
It is better to let it last for many years;
and to anchor at the island when you are old,
rich with all you have gained on the way . . .
Ithaca has given you the beautiful voyage.
Without her you would have never set out on the road.

From Ithaca by Cavanfy (1863–1933), (Sachperoglou, 2007, p. 37)

When the editing team began to compile this book, we were struck by the similarity of our own experiences of working, teaching and learning to use problem-based learning (PBL) and the metaphor of a journey. As educators, we were aware that our own journeys travelled paths both well worn on occasions and exciting, fresh and ever surprising at the same time. Despite the numerous questions that can be asked when working with and through PBL, part of the essence of the work is the journey of learning. The student and educator move together into the unknown, learning with a freedom of discovery. This keeps us engaged on that road with curiosity and in search of answers and truths, wherever and whatever they may be. The energy for PBL felt strongly by the writing team derives from the value placed on that educational journey. We felt that this was an important text to write because although PBL is an empowering way of working, paradoxically, by taking away familiar structures of traditional education, many people struggle and can feel de-skilled when first encountering it, either as a student or as an educator. We hope this text will therefore help provide a positive way into this work, helping people understand and engage in the fullest potential of the journey and benefiting from what it can offer. This is because PBL can be a pivotal experience enabling students to drive confidently into a world where their skill and ability as self-motivated lifelong learners is essential to develop ever-growing expertise in practice. For readers with more experience of PBL, we hope the book will present challenging ideas and provoke further consideration of contemporary practice as well as a revisiting of more familiar ideas.

For the contributors to this book, this process has included reflecting on the real-world practicalities of working this way in higher education settings, revisiting and developing the theory that guides a contemporary use of PBL, and examining the curriculum experience for both the learner and the educator. The experience of the contributors is based mainly (although not exclusively) in higher education settings for health and social care professionals, and inevitably that experience has influenced our approach to the writing. Collectively, we have come to PBL in different ways – as students enrolled on this style of course, as staff working on a programme using PBL or as course designers who have actively elected to construct a curriculum with this method of teaching and learning. We hope this book will appeal not only to colleagues and students in the health and social care sector but also to other professional groups using PBL or thinking of adopting it within teaching and learning.

As with any text informed by experience, a number of themes were identified as important by the writing team and these are reflected within various chapters of the text. As themes emerged, were debated and then revised for this publication, a logical shape emerged from the writing that led to the development of three sections or parts to structure the approach taken by contributors. Each of these parts is a distinct entity with a convergence of focus shared by that group of writers, possibly helping readers to find material of interest in a convenient way. In turn, each part links to and complements the others within the book, building up a collection of writing from different perspectives on PBL that are both interlinked and yet distinct in their focus. In addition to the three structural parts, there is this introductory chapter to help navigate the reader into the text and a final concluding chapter in Part 3, written by Teena J. Clouston.

Part 1 – 'General Principles of Using PBL' – examines some key areas of common concern to all people engaged in using this way of teaching and learning, such as in Chapter 2, which explores some of the history of PBL and its relevance to curricula today. This said, some chapters may be of particular interest to educators seeking to introduce PBL into their educational practice or critically examine and develop their expertise in this area. There are chapters that prompt the reader to carefully consider whether the time is right to switch to this type of learning as well as those that explore a wide range of practical and theoretical concepts that enable PBL to be practised in a thoughtful and effective way. The titles of chapters in Part 1 are as follows:

Chapter 2: Exploring the foundations for problem-based learning – Ruth Matheson and Bernhard Haas

Chapter 3: Readiness for problem-based learning – Juan Delport and Steven W. Whitcombe

Chapter 4: Developing problem-based learning curricula – Lyn Westcott, Alison Seymour and Sara Roberts

Chapter 5: Becoming a problem-based learning facilitator – Gwilym Wyn Roberts

Chapter 6: Managing group dynamics and developing team working in problem-based learning – Alison Seymour

Chapter 7: Assessing problem-based learning curricula – Sue Pengelly

Part 2 – 'The Theoretical Interface with PBL' – is designed to explore in some depth a selection of theoretical constructs and concepts, offering established and newer discussion on how PBL may be framed and practised. Informed by a body of primary research into these topics, the chapters in this part aim to develop and consolidate the work of other writers and theorists in this area. The key feature of their approach is that they also offer some different emergent insights on the relevance of a particular theory for the practice of PBL. The work will be of interest to readers who wish to explore theoretical parameters alongside some areas of topical debate and reasoning. These chapters and this part of the book are not definitive in their scope, but offer some debate that is different from that found in other PBL texts. It is hoped that they will engage PBL practitioners in discussion on how this work may be further developed and applied. The titles of chapters in Part 2 are as follows:

Chapter 8: Reflection and the problem-based learning curriculum – Gail Boniface

Chapter 9: A reflexive model for problem-based learning – Steven W. Whitcombe and Teena J. Clouston

Chapter 10: Promoting creative thinking and innovative practice through the use of problem-based learning – Jill Riley and Ruth Matheson

Chapter 11: Problem-based learning and the development of capital – Jill Riley and Steven W. Whitcombe

Chapter 12: An evolving vision for learning in health-care education – Andrew Machon and Gwilym Wyn Roberts

Part 3 – 'The Learner in Problem-Based Learning' – is a section that explores relevant dimensions for students using PBL as part of their passage to professional practice and beyond. The work discusses some frank first-hand experience of the student journey, as well as examining a selection of critical interrelated issues when using PBL during study for health and social care professions. This is considered as part of a wider remit of becoming a lifelong learner as well as a qualified practitioner. The work will be of interest not only to health and social care students using PBL but also to other students whose curricula include this type of learning experience. The chapters will also be useful to educators – either those beginning to work in a curriculum using PBL or more experienced staff seeking to appreciate more about the potential of PBL as part of the student journey and about how this contributes to development of professionally responsible practitioners in health and social care. The following are the titles of chapters in Part 3:

Chapter 13: The student experience – Liz Galle and Sandra Marshman

Chapter 14: Becoming lifelong learners in health and social care – Pam Stead, Gareth Morgan and Sally Scott-Roberts

Chapter 15: Becoming a self-directed learner – Susan Delport and Ruth Squire

In the final Part 4 of the book, strands of thinking in problem-based learning have been interweaved by Teena J. Clouston under 'Final Thoughts'. This highlights some conclusions in the light of the content of the book and discusses an interconnected, relational perspective for PBL.

As a group we have been interested in reflecting on our educational experience and understanding of PBL derived from notable contributors in this area relevant to our own practice, including Boud and Feletti (1997), Engel (1997), Baptiste (2003), Sadlo and Richardson (2003) and Savin-Baden (2000, 2003). Some writers have drawn on PBL as an area for conceptual analysis within their higher studies and all have engaged in lively debates with peers and colleagues. This has enabled us to develop our understanding, challenge the ethos and direction of practice as well as consolidate ideas contributing to and shaping the work at hand. We hope that our presentation of some of these areas within this book will appeal both to those new to and those familiar with PBL. As a group we are aware that there is a divergence of opinion on aspects of PBL and enquiry-based learning and how these may be drawn upon within a curriculum. The remit of this text is not broad enough to explore all this in depth, but it does include aspects of opinion that may explore ways forward, challenge understanding and address theory and practice issues topical and familiar to people within the PBL community. We hope that the book will inspire further debate and help engage even more people into this way of working. We are still on our personal roads to Ithaca; let us enjoy the adventure and knowledge that unfolds ahead.

References

Baptiste, S. (2003) *Problem-Based Learning: A Self-Directed Journey*. Slack Incorporated, Thorofare, NJ.

Boud, D. & Feletti, G. (1997) *The Challenge of Problem-Based Learning*, 2nd edn. Kogan Page, London.

Engel, C. (1997) Not just a method but a way of learning. In: *The Challenge of Problem-Based Learning* (eds D. Boud & G. Feletti). Kogan Page, London.

Sachperoglou, E. (2007) *CP Cavanfy The Collected Poems: A New Translation. Oxford World Classics*. Oxford University Press, Oxford.

Sadlo, G. & Richardson, J.T.E. (2003) Approaches to studying and perceptions of the academic environment in students following problem based learning and subject based curricula. *Higher Education Research and Development*. **22** (3), 253–274.

Savin-Baden, M. (2000) *Problem-Based Learning in Higher Education: Untold Stories*. Open University Press, Maidenhead.

Savin-Baden, M. (2003) *Facilitating Problem-Based Learning: Illuminating Perspectives*. Open University Press, Maidenhead.

Part 1

General Principles of Using Problem-Based Learning

2: Exploring the foundations for problem-based learning

Ruth Matheson and Bernhard Haas

Introduction

This chapter provides the reader with a foundation for understanding the evolution of problem-based learning (PBL) from its beginning to current thinking on the same. It begins with a definition of PBL and considers why this is an appropriate approach for the education of health and social care professionals. It seeks to link the aims and objectives of PBL programmes with the development of skills necessary to function in a modern health and social care environment. Examples of two different models of PBL have been provided to show a comparison between the well-publicised Seven Step Maastricht Model and a less procedural visual model, both demonstrating the cyclical nature of the PBL process. The chapter proceeds to provide insight into the links between PBL with both the principles of adult education, as presented by Knowles (1980), and current educational thinking regarding the constructive nature of learning. The final section examines both the advantages and disadvantages of PBL as presented in the literature, while challenging the reader to consider the benefits of the adoption of PBL by health and social care educational programmes.

Definition of problem-based learning

A basic definition for PBL is provided by Boud and Feletti (1997, p. 15), which describes it as 'an approach to structuring the curriculum which involves confronting students with problems from practice which provide a stimulus for learning'. Boud and Feletti, however, also acknowledge that this definition could be applied to other learning approaches. The essential delineating characteristic of PBL is that learning is initiated by the learners' focus on problem resolution without propositional knowledge (Savin-Baden, 2000). 'Real-life' problems provide the initial impetus to promote exploration of the problem and to begin the process of critical thinking. By working in small groups, utilising their collective skills, students develop collaborative processes to identify individual and group learning needs in order to solve the problem. Individual research informs the group, and through interrogation and integration of the information, understanding is developed and used to provide potential solutions and identify further needs. The process of learning is active, self-directed and cyclical.

Why adopt a problem-based learning approach in health and social care?

Educators in health and social care have been inspired to adopt a PBL approach for their courses for a number of reasons. The growth and development of PBL has gone hand in hand with the rapid expansion in biomedical knowledge, and Epstein (2004) proposed that more traditional, didactic methods are unable to cope with teaching this vast increase in factual knowledge. Priorities are shifting from merely acquiring knowledge to providing the learner and developing professional with the skills for lifelong learning. Health and social care professions are seen essentially as practice-based disciplines. The clinical education/ placement element of education programmes often fulfil the crucial task in linking university-based theoretical education and clinical/ professional and practice education. It has been widely accepted that not all education programmes successfully make this link (Tiwari *et al.*, 2006). The creation of positive learning contexts that help to bridge this theory/practice gap is therefore essential. This learning context plays a vital role in developing appropriate learning behaviour. Deep learning is seen as a positive and appropriate approach for students to adopt as it will help them to accumulate knowledge and, at the same time, to apply it to the situations faced in everyday practice. Surface learning, on the other hand, is seen as inappropriate as it merely relies on memorisation and does not facilitate understanding and reflective application. The use of real-life scenarios in PBL aims to provide this essential context for learning. Schmidt (1983) describes PBL as an instructional method that presents a small group of students with a carefully constructed problem reflecting real-life phenomena. This problem needs exploration; through discussion students find explanations and seek ways to solve the problem presented (Schmidt, 1983). Once learning objectives have been established, further individual learning is needed to inform the group of knowledge, understanding and insights that will assist in the resolution of the problem. Barrows and Tamlyn (1980) highlight the need to gain this knowledge from a variety of external sources and develop the ability to integrate information gained to solve the problem, thereby integrating theory and practice.

Health and social care practitioners cannot only rely on acquiring knowledge and practical skills, even if they are equipped to update these in line with new developments. Modern health and social care needs individuals who are good at team working, coping with change and uncertainty, solving problems and making reasoned decisions (Hmelo & Evensen, 2000).

Aims and objectives of PBL programmes

The aims of PBL and the outcomes by which any successful PBL programme should be judged (summarised from Barrows, 1994; Newman, 2003) are listed below.

- Acquisition of integrated, applied and extensive knowledge
- Development of independent, self-directed lifelong learning skills
- Development of practical, professional and interpersonal skills
- Development of motivation to learn, question and understand
- Early immersion into the culture and values of health and social care and professional attitude
- Development of collaboration and team working skills
- Ability to adapt to and participate in change
- Problem solving and making reasoned decisions in unfamiliar situations
- Reasoning critically and creatively
- Practising with empathy, appreciating the other person's point of view

Not all PBL programmes achieve all of these objectives all of the time for all learners. However, there are strong claims that PBL is good at developing these interpersonal skills (Spronken-Smith, 2005) and that it prepares the learners well for their professional roles (Jones *et al.*, 2002; Dean *et al.*, 2003).

Central to PBL is the student-centred approach. The student-centred nature of the learning reflects the principles of adult learning set out by Knowles (1980), recognising the need for adult learners to be perceived and treated by others as being capable of taking responsibility for themselves, coming to the learning environment with a wealth of experience and learning what they need to know in order to perform effectively; it also recognises that for learning to be meaningful it needs to be centred around life situations and not subject matter (Knowles, 1980, 1984).

Barrows (1994) identifies the brainstorming stage of the PBL process as the beginning of the clinical reasoning process. He suggests that the generation of multiple hypotheses results in a creative aspect of problem solving that requires the students to think laterally about the problem, producing new and unique ideas to be explored. It is from the exploration of these hypotheses that learning needs develop and the knowledge needed to test out the hypotheses can be identified. Having gained and analysed the knowledge in relation to the hypotheses (independent study and research), it is time for the students to share their ideas and findings with the group to hone the ideas presented and judgments made (feedback and discussion) in order to make a final group decision and evaluate the outcome (action and evaluation).

Student centredness also means that learning is motivating, challenging and rewarding. PBL students certainly seem to have more fun (Dolmans & Schmidt, 1996) and rate their educational experiences higher than those from more traditional courses (Smits *et al.*, 2002). They also seem to have a better retention through their PBL courses and demonstrate a better progression into post-graduate education (Susarla *et al.*, 2003).

Chronology of problem-based learning

The idea of PBL is certainly not a new one. The approach originated in medical education in the 1960s at McMaster University in Canada. The basis for its introduction was a large-scale dissatisfaction with traditional lecture-based teaching, which appeared to be promoting fact-based rote learning. Out of this dissatisfaction grew problem-based learning (PBL). To date, PBL has probably been applied in one form or another in most medical schools in the United States. Dental schools were somewhat slower to adopt the approach. PBL has also been introduced in many medical schools in the United Kingdom. Other programmes in health and social care have also embraced the approach and the Department of Health (1999) has encouraged its adoption in nursing, midwifery and health visiting education. PBL has also been embraced by subjects outside the medical, health and social care arena. There are recent positive examples from geography (Spronken-Smith, 2005) and business management (Kanet & Barut, 2003), to name but two.

The implementation of PBL is certainly not uniform, and this variability makes its evaluation a considerable challenge. Some programmes may restrict PBL to certain elements of the overall curriculum. For example, PBL may be applied to the more theoretical or university-based elements or modules of a health programme without its implementation in placement. Others have specifically focused on PBL in the clinical/placement element of learning (Tiwari *et al.*, 2006; Ehrenberg & Haeggblom, 2007).

Many forms and variations of PBL exist today and the relative merit of 'pure' versus 'hybrid' forms is probably impossible to answer with a high degree of confidence. This is largely due to the fact that published evaluations or comparisons usually fail to adequately describe the PBL or the control approach taken. A clear definition of 'what is hybrid PBL' is lacking, but Armstrong (1997) explains it as 'innovation without sacrificing the best of the old'. In practice, this would often involve a problem-focused approach, combined with the retention of lectures and skills classes. This form of PBL is often adopted by health and social care programmes as they seek to ensure competency of skills and satisfy regulatory body requirements. It could be argued that this approach also provides students with a greater sense of security in their foundation knowledge and skills for practice and mirrors the type of experience gained while on clinical practice.

Common to most PBL approaches is the attempt to provide a clear structure (McLoughlin & Darvill, 2007). This structure commonly involves the use of a trigger or case scenario. This trigger may be taken from real practice or be adapted from real practice with the intention to better cover the intended outcomes of learning. The learners then have to develop their own learning objectives, drawing on existing knowledge and defining new learning needs (Wood, 2003). The learners then work on these objectives before they share their findings with the other group members. While this PBL structure is the key to the development and achievement of the learner, it is frequently supplemented with other sessions. These can be practical skills classes, clinical practice on placements, keynote lectures or other resource sessions (Wood, 2003). What differentiates PBL from other types of group learning is its focus on problem resolution from the outset, irrespective of propositional knowledge.

Models of problem-based learning

A number of models for this PBL process have been described and are in use. Probably the best known and most widely used of these models is the Maastricht Seven Step Model (Schmidt, 1983) described below:

Step 1: Clarifying the text and explaining unclear terms and concepts

Students are presented with the problem, they read through the text and identify any concepts or words that are unclear to ensure a joint group understanding.

Step 2: Defining the key problem

The students work together to define the problem or identify the key task.

Step 3: Analysing the problem and suggesting possible solutions

This is the brainstorming stage where ideas are presented as to what may be causing the problem. At this stage no idea should be thrown out or sifted and students should discuss their understanding of the problem from their particular standpoint and offer possible solutions.

Step 4: Elaborating, testing, reviewing and refining

The group discusses the ideas put forward in Step 3 and the students begin to prioritise their findings. It is at this stage that they remove any irrelevant information. Any possible solutions should be recorded and discussions should ensue to prioritise these.

Step 5: Formulating learning objectives

A group consensus is reached with regard to the sound knowledge base needed to address the problem. Learning needs are identified and prioritised by establishing what the group does not know or understand and by establishing how these needs can be met. It is at this stage that a group learning contract can be useful (Matheson, 2003).

Step 6: Self-study

Students research individually to gain information about their learning objectives. Encouragement should be given to obtain this information from a variety of sources including books, journal and personal contacts.

Step 7: Integrating and testing new information

The individual research is brought back to the group. The knowledge and understanding needs to be synthesised to present its relevance to the problem and, through discussion/debate, scrutinised in relation to the problem. Following feedback, the group may need to return to Step 2 to redefine the problem and the process starts again.

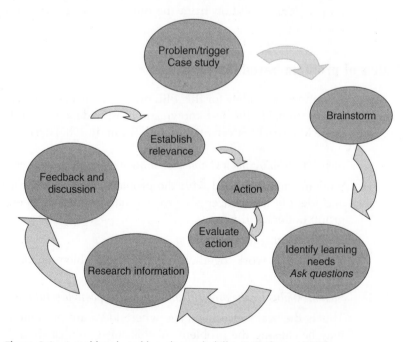

Figure 2.1 A problem-based learning cycle (Riley & Matheson, 2005).

The use of a model provides students with a structure and potential sense of security especially in the initial stages of learning to adopt this style of learning. However, the rigid nature of following the process step by step can be restrictive and may not allow for deviation and may potentially inhibit creativity.

Other less rigid models of PBL have been developed which provide students with a process but demand a less structured approach. In all these cases, the process is cyclical, with the facilitator helping students learn the cognitive skills necessary for problem solving and collaboration (Hmelo-Silver, 2004). One such model, represented in a visual form (Figure 2.1), has been developed as a result of research by Riley and Matheson (2005), linked in Chapter 10 to the creative analytical framework.

An informed and rounded discussion of PBL must include a review of its theoretical basis in educational psychology and adult learning.

Problem-based learning and its links with adult learners

In determining whether to pursue the adoption of PBL, it is important to have an understanding of the principles of adult learning and to identify how PBL meets these needs. In 1980, Knowles set out his principles of adult learning, organising his findings into a model to be later revised in 1998, to incorporate further insights gained into factors that affect adult learning.

Knowles *et al.* (1998a,b, p. 4) identified the core principles of adult learning as follows:

■ Self-concept of the learner
■ Prior experience of the learner
■ Readiness to learn
■ Orientation to learning
■ Motivation to learn

To these core principles they added two dimensions: goals and purpose for learning; individual and situational differences.

In order to establish how these relate to PBL, we need to demonstrate the links and identify how these affect practice. This is particularly pertinent to health and social care where learning should centre on a person-centred approach.

Within PBL, students identify their own learning needs, establish what they should investigate, justify why they should pursue the line of enquiry and establish how, as individuals, they might go about gaining appropriate knowledge. This 'need to know' is one of the factors that led McMaster University to adopt PBL, wanting their students to integrate knowledge and be able to understand why a piece of knowledge was necessary to understand an individual problem. Linderman (1926), one of the founders of the principles of adult learning, identified that adults are motivated to learn when they experience a need and lack knowledge to satisfy their interest. In identifying both group and individual needs, the students within PBL groups seek to satisfy their own curiosity and work collaboratively to provide a knowledge base. This, once synthesised, will offer potential solutions to the problems. Knowles *et al.* (2005, p. 65) stress the need for facilitators to learning to help learners become aware of the 'need to know'. This can be achieved through the skills of the facilitator. The influence of the facilitator on the learning in PBL has been discussed by a number of authors (Groves *et al.*, 2005; Van Berkel & Dolmans, 2006) and will be addressed further in Chapter 5.

Knowles *et al.* (2005) describe the self-concept of the adult learner as being autonomous and self-directing. The need to enhance the students' ability to be self-directed is at the heart of PBL and requires appropriate curriculum design in the early stages of a PBL course to develop these skills. It is vitally important that students are given opportunities to take control of their learning and identify their own learning needs. This is particularly important for those leaving the school environment where they have been conditioned to be dependent on the teacher. This transition to self-directedness needs to be inherent from the outset, with learners being viewed as being capable of making their own decision and choosing their own direction. This can be difficult to achieve within health and social care programmes with set requirements from professional bodies regarding the content of curricula design and set learning outcomes to be achieved to meet regulatory standards. These constraints often produce conflict between content (knowledge and skills) that can be seen as essential to meet professional standards and the need to allow learners the autonomy to determine their own content, driven by a need to know, taking into account prior experience.

Adults come to the learning environment with experience and therefore they become a resource for others' learning. It is this experience that adds to the richness of the PBL discussion and helps to provide the integration of theory and practice. However, this experience also has the potential for the creation of conflict as learners may come with fixed ideas and be less open to differing points of view. This is a challenge for the group members in learning to handle difficult individuals and for the tutor to facilitate thinking outside of the individual's lived experiences while not undervaluing their views. Coming from different backgrounds, cultures, experiences, needs and having different motivations means that there is a need to provide a more individualised learning and teaching experience (Knowles *et al.*, 2005).

By drawing on these different experiences and prompting consideration of different scenarios (Chapter 10), the facilitator can challenge the students to explore other possibilities and challenge their own potentially rigid views.

Knowles (1980) proposes that individuals come with a readiness to learn what they need to know in order to deal with a given situation. Although students come with a readiness to learn, their previous educational experience may not have prepared them for the challenges of higher education, in particular, PBL. Therefore, there is a need to support students, particularly in the early stages of this developmental process. This may require curricula design to recognise the need to be developmental in nature, a fact that supports the development of the spiral curriculum (Chapter 4). The development of skills needs to be incremental in nature and may need to be introduced through alternative activities that scaffold the PBL process (e.g. skills-based workshops, experiential learning and simulations).

Adults' orientation to learning is life centred, whereas children's learning focuses on subject-based material. This is particularly relevant for PBL as problems/triggers centre around scenarios that require groups and individuals to develop skills, knowledge and strategies to address real-life issues, tasks or problems, thereby making learning relevant and meaningful.

In 1998, Knowles *et al.* added two additional dimensions to their model: Goals and Purposes for Learning, and Individual and Situational Differences. The goals and purposes describe the missions of the adult education (Knowles *et al.*, 2005). These are for individual, institutional or societal growth and are the outcomes of the learning. The individual and situational differences recognise that subject matter may need to be dealt with by different learning strategies; for example, if a technical skill is to be learnt then self-directed learning may not be the best vehicle for this and a more behavioural approach may be more appropriate; likewise, situations may determine the style of learning adopted, for example, the size of the groups. Learners' individual differences may require unique learning programmes to be developed to meet individuals' needs. Once again, this forces us to recognise the potential need to move away from the purest form of PBL to establish whether other learning and teaching styles need to be incorporated to address the needs of learners and, in particular, meet the needs of modern health and social care professionals.

Problem-based learning and its links with modern learning

Modern insights into learning have tended to focus on a constructivist viewpoint, which will be explored by looking at the concepts and linking these with the process of PBL.

Dolmans *et al.* (2005, p. 732) state that PBL reflects modern insights into learning:

> Modern insights into learning emphasise that learning should be a constructive, self-directed, collaborative and contextual process

It is these four elements of modern learning that will be discussed in relation to the theory and practice of PBL.

- Learning should be a constructive process based on prior knowledge.
- Learners should be self-directed and self-evaluative.
- Learning is a collaborative process.
- Learning should be placed in a clear context.

Constructive process

In order for learning to take place there needs to be an active process within the students to construct or reconstruct their knowledge networks and learn to build their own interpretations. In other words, students come to the learning environment with prior knowledge, which, they will re-evaluate, in the light of new insights gained, and reconstruct to incorporate their new ideas, insights and understanding. The challenge for educators in developing PBL curriculum is the need to develop learning opportunities that allow students from diverse backgrounds and with different life experiences to feel that they have something to contribute from the start. It is therefore vitally important then that the case studies/triggers used to stimulate learning have relevance to the students and are clearly rooted in real-life scenarios while providing opportunities to approach the problem using new insights gained (Chapter 10). These insights are achieved by the process of elaboration through questioning, challenging perceptions and discussion, helping the student to make links between concepts and forming relationships between knowledge and practice, thereby making better use of the knowledge gained. Facilitation of the groups should focus on assisting students to develop the skills of elaboration and should be recognised as being developmental in nature (Chapter 5).

Self-directed process

Self-directed learning involves the learners taking an active role in their learning process. This involves learners, from the outset, planning what their learning needs are, to address a given problem. This means that learners within a group will approach a problem from very different positions, depending on their prior experience, existing knowledge base and personal approach. What is important in being self-directed is that the learning environment allows for and encourages these differences and that diversity of opinion is seen as enriching to the group. This requires problems to be developed that do not lead the learner to a foregone conclusion, but are complex enough to motivate the learner and provide opportunities for decision-making and critical thinking. For the individuals, the challenge of becoming self-directed is to develop the skills to plan, monitor and evaluate their learning (Dolmans *et al.*, 2005). A useful tool to aid this development and assist in recognising learning needs, resources and assist in the self-monitoring and evaluation is a learning contract. The learning contract helps to make the learning less ambiguous and assists in the planning stage in particular, and can be used both on an individual and a group basis (Matheson, 2003). Another useful tool in helping learners recognise their readiness for this process is through the use of the reflexive model for PBL discussed in Chapter 9. Motivation is key to the promotion of self-directed learning and therefore the relevance of learning to future practice must be clearly evident if the learner is to remain engaged.

Collaborative process

One of the dangers of PBL is that the group subdivides work in order to complete the task. This can become the case when the group is driven by completion of a task rather than concentrating on the learning process and a number of possible solutions. Groups must have a common goal and share the responsibility for resolving the problem, be mutually dependent and value each other's input. This is difficult to achieve in a group where individuals have different drives and where task-orientated individuals exist. A clear message needs to be provided from the outset that the value of PBL lies in the process as much as in the outcome. In order for this collaboration to take place, students need to feel at ease with each other both socially and cognitively, and be supportive with an expectation that all members will participate. Time needs to be taken in preparing learners for group work, and part of the facilitation process is concerned with creating a safe environment to allow questioning and challenging. Examining roles taken within groups, regular peer evaluation built into the group sessions, feedback on group performance and learning how to challenge assist in the development of these skills. Consideration needs to be given to the length of tutorials, allowing time for discussion rather than just the division of labour. Recent research found that group cohesiveness and culture were the major contributing factors to students' withdrawal from participation and decreased motivation (discussed in Chapter 6).

Contextual process

One of the insights of modern learning is the need for learning to be placed within a context. This is particularly important when using PBL, as the problem will vary depending on the context in which it is placed.

Given the need for real-life scenarios, this becomes even more evident. Dolmans *et al.* (2005) highlight that viewing problem environments from multiple perspectives increases transfer of knowledge. One way of providing this multiple perspective is through the use of a spiral curriculum (Chapter 4) through which the learners revisit knowledge at an increasing depth from differing contexts, having to utilise their previous learning and reconstructing it to examine another situation. This revisiting also helps to promote reflective practice, drawing on previous experience to be examined in the light of new circumstances. The type of triggers presented to the learner appears to have a major impact on the type of learning activity that is undertaken. Those triggers presenting a narrative account lead learners to look for clues, whereas ill-defined problems lead to demands for decision-making and action (Lloyd-Jones *et al.*, 1998). The nature of these triggers will be further discussed in the chapter on creativity (Chapter 10). Once again the importance of ensuring professional relevance is paramount.

Historically, tutor facilitation within PBL has viewed the role of the tutor as one of passive observer inputting into the group to ensure clarity of the trigger and questioning to ensure a depth of understanding and to elicit a deeper learning. It has been suggested that tutors/facilitators do not have to have detailed knowledge of the subject area in order to facilitate PBL groups. However, modern insights into learning have highlighted the need for tutors to be more active in their role as facilitators.

Dolmans *et al.* (2005) view the tutor's role as that of supporting student learning by stimulating discussion, providing stimulus for elaboration, encouraging the integration of knowledge and promoting interaction between students. They see this as being achieved through asking questions, seeking clarification and providing insights to enhance the application of knowledge.

The benefits/limitations of problem-based learning

PBL has many supporters who cite its many achievements and advantages over more traditional teaching methods. The following provides some examples but is by no means intended to be an exhaustive review.

PBL has been found to be more effective than traditional methods in developing lifelong learning skills and perceived to be a more enjoyable way of learning (Dolmans & Schmidt, 1996). This increased motivation and enjoyment is not just restricted to the students but it also affects their educators and facilitators (Colliver, 2000). Learning behaviour, with improved self-directed learning skills, was reported by Williams in 1999 in a study involving nursing students who had been exposed to PBL. Tiwari *et al.* (2006) found that a significantly deeper learning approach had occurred as a consequence of exposure to

PBL experiences while on placement. Spronken-Smith (2005) described the well-developed transferable skills, particularly team working. PBL students showed significantly better learning behaviour in terms of learning self-regulation and a more constructive concept of learning. The students felt that they were more active contributors to the learning process (Lycke *et al.*, 2006). In a study involving dental students (Susarla *et al.*, 2003), it was found that the introduction of the PBL approach led to an improvement in exam results, compared to previous intakes of students who had been exposed to a traditional lecture-based programme. The readiness and preparedness for practice of their medical students was investigated by Dean *et al.* (2003) and also by Jones *et al.* (2002). They found that their graduates felt, on the whole, more prepared for practice and also more confident in areas such as interpersonal skills, confidence, collaboration, holistic care and self-directed learning.

PBL certainly also has its critics who, on the whole, feel that claims for its superiority may be overstated and cannot be supported by clear evidence. Colliver (2000) suggested that PBL students do not appear to produce significantly better examination results than students from more traditional programmes. He bases this on what he describes as a lack of size effect and clearly reported similarities between PBL and non-PBL students. He therefore cautions that widespread change to PBL curricula in medicine with its potentially increased resource demands may not be justified. Colliver's disappointment in his perceived lack of measurable superiority of PBL students also implies that PBL students are in many areas at least as good as non-PBL students. A common area of concern is the ability to acquire factual knowledge. In challenging Colliver's pessimism, Norman and Schmidt (2000) summarise the research as follows: PBL students perform in a manner similar to non-PBL students on examination results, suggesting comparable levels of knowledge acquisition but a potential for better knowledge retention. There are small differences in the learning of clinical skills for PBL students and consistent reports of better satisfaction with their learning. The evidence base for PBL certainly has been challenged by Colliver (2000) and methodological weaknesses in the literature cannot be denied.

Conclusions

PBL is an exciting way to facilitate learning in health and social care. A number of different professions and health-care programmes have successfully adopted this approach. PBL is firmly based on an understanding of current learning theories of adult learning and PBL will enable the learners to acquire the necessary knowledge that forms the basis of their professional practice. Research has shown that knowledge acquisition in PBL is at least as good as in more traditional teaching settings. What makes PBL different is the emphasis on the presentation of an initial problem without the pre-delivery of knowledge. PBL therefore focuses not just on the acquisition of knowledge but places a high importance on the development of communication skills, team skills and lifelong learning skills. Anyone working in health and social care will appreciate that these are key skills and competences of a modern professional.

PBL should not be confused with 'problem solving', although it will greatly enhance the ability of the learner to improve their problem-solving skills. Savin-Baden (2000) differentiates between problem-solving learning and PBL, stating that the two are often confused with each other. Problem-solving learning is used across many disciplines and requires students to problem solve, having been provided with the necessary prerequisite knowledge. Many programmes in health and social care will utilise forms of problem solving within their curricula. What makes PBL different is that the learning starts from the problem and that knowledge and skills are developed out of recognition of what is necessary to solve the problem. This aim of PBL is to develop professional insight (Biggs & Tang, 2007) and to prepare the learner for immediate post qualification entry into the workforce. Anyone who is considering the adoption of this approach to their profession or programme is encouraged to do so. Many others have successfully made the transition already.

References

Armstrong, E.G. (1997) A hybrid model of problem-based learning. In: *The Challenge of Problem Based Learning* (eds D. Boud & G. Feletti), pp. 137–151. Kogan Page, London.

Barrows, H.S. (1994) *Problem-Based Learning Applied to Medical Education*. Southern Illinois University School of Medicine, IL.

Barrows, H.S. & Tamlyn, R.M. (1980) *Problem-Based Learning: An Approach to Medical Education*. Springer Publishing Company, New York, NY.

Biggs, J. & Tang, C. (2007) *Teaching for Quality at University*, 3rd edn. Society for Research into Higher Education/Open University Press, Buckingham.

Boud, D. & Feletti, G. (1997) Part 1: what is problem-based learning? In: *The Challenge of Problem-Based Learning* (eds D. Boud & G. Felleti), pp. 15–16. Kogan Page, London.

Colliver, J.A. (2000) Effectiveness of problem-based learning curricula: research and theory. *Academic Medicine.* **75** (3), 59–266.

Dean, S.J., Barratt, A.L., Hendry, G.D. & Lyon, P.M.A. (2003) Preparedness for hospital practice among graduates of a problem-based, graduate-entry medical program. *Medical Journal of Australia.* **178**, 163–167.

Department of Health (1999) *Making a Difference: Strengthening the Nursing, Midwifery and Health Visiting Contribution to Health and Healthcare*. Department of Health, Crown Publications, London.

Dolmans, D. & Schmidt, H.G. (1996) The advantages of problem-based curricula. *Postgraduate Medical Journal*. **72**, 535–538.

Dolmans, D.H., De Grave, W.S., Wolfhagen, I.H.A.P. & van der Vleuten, C.P. (2005) Problem-based learning: future challenges for educational practice and research. *Medical Education*. **39**, 732–741.

Ehrenberg, A.C. & Haeggblom, M. (2007) Problem-based learning in clinical nursing education: integrating theory and practice. *Nurse Education in Practice*. **7**, 67–74.

Epstein, R.J. (2004) Learning from the problems of problem-based learning. *BMC Medical Education*. **4**, 1. Available at: http://www.biomedcentral.com/1472-6920/4/1. Accessed on 27th July 2009.

Groves, M., Rego, P. & O'Rourke, P. (2005) Tutoring in problem-based learning medical curricula: the influence of tutor background and style on effectiveness. *BMC Medical Education*. **5**, 20. Available at: http://www.biomedcentral.com/1472-6920/5/20. Accessed on 27th July 2009.

Hmelo, C.E. & Evensen, D.H. (2000) Introduction: problem-based learning: gaining insights on learning interactions through multiple methods of Inquiry. In: *Problem-Based Learning: A Research Perspective on Learning Interactions* (eds D.H. Evensen & C.E. Hmelo), pp. 1–19. Lawrence Erlbaum Associates, NJ.

Hmelo-Silver, C.E. (2004) Problem-based learning: what and how do students learn? *Educational Psychology Review*. **16** (3), 235–265.

Jones, A., McArdle, P.J. & O'Neill, P.A. (2002) Perceptions of how well graduates are prepared for the role of pre-registration house officer: a comparison of outcomes from a traditional and an integrated PBL curriculum. *Medical Education*. **36**, 16–25.

Kanet, J.J. & Barut, M. (2003) Problem-based learning for production and operations management. *Decision Sciences Journal of Innovative Education*. **1** (1), 99–118.

Knowles, M., Holton, E. & Swanson, R. (1998a) *The Adult Learner; The Definitive in Adult Education and Human Resource Development*, 5th edn. Elsevier, London.

Knowles, M., Holton, E. & Swanson, R. (1998b) *The Adult Learner; The Definitive in Adult Education and Human Resource Development*, 6th edn. Elsevier, London.

Knowles, M.S., Holton, E.F. & Swanson, R. (2005) *The Adult Learner*, 6th edn. Elsevier, London.

Knowles, M.S. (1980) *The Modern Practice of Adult Education. From Pedagogy to Andragogy*, 2nd edn. Follet, Chicago, IL.

Knowles, M.S. (1984) *Andragogy in Action: Applying Modern Principles of Adult Learning*. Jossey-Bass Inc., San Francisco, CA.

Linderman, E.C. (1926) *The Meaning of Adult Education*. Republic Inc., New York, NY.

Lloyd-Jones, G., Margetson, D. & Bligh, J.G. (1998) Problem-based learning: a coat of many colours. *Medical Education*. **32**, 492–494.

Lycke, K.H., Grottom, P. & Stromso, H.I. (2006) Student learning strategies, mental models and learning outcomes in problem-based and traditional curricula in medicine. *Medical Teacher*. **28** (8), 717–722.

Matheson, R.M. (2003) Promoting the integration of theory and practice by the use of a learning contract. *International Journal of Therapy and Rehabilitation*. **10** (6), 264–269.

McLoughlin, M. & Darvill, A. (2007) Peeling back the layers of learning: a classroom model for problem-based learning. *Nurse Education Today*. **27**, 271–277.

Newman, M. (2003) *A Pilot Systematic Review and Meta Analysis on the Effectiveness of Problem Based Learning – Special Report 2*. Learning and Teaching Support Network Subject Centre for Medicine, Dentistry and Veterinary Medicine, Newcastle (ISBN: 0701701587).

Norman, G.R. & Schmidt, H.G. (2000) Effectiveness of problem based learning curricula: theory, practice and paper darts. *Medical Education*. **34**, 721–728.

Riley, J. & Matheson, R. (2005). Enhancing students' creativity through problem-based learning: a challenge for curriculum design. *International Conference on Problem-Based Learning: Lahti, Finland* (May 2005). Paper Presentation.

Savin-Baden, M. (2000) *Problem-Based Learning in Higher Education: Untold Stories*. Society for Research into Higher Education/Open University Press, Buckingham.

Schmidt, H.G. (1983) Problem based learning: rationale and description. *Medical Education*. **17**, 11–16.

Smits, P.B.A., Verbeek, J.H.A.M. & De Buisonje, C.D. (2002) Problem based learning in continuing medical education: a review of controlled evaluation studies. *British Medical Journal*. **324**, 153–156.

Spronken-Smith, R. (2005) Implementing a problem-based learning approach for teaching research methods in geography. *Journal of Geography in Higher Education*. **29** (2), 203–221.

Susarla, S.M., Medina-Martinez, N., Howell, T.H. & Karimbux, N.Y. (2003) Problem-based learning: effects on standard outcomes. *Journal of Dental Education*. **67** (9), 1003–1010.

Tiwari, A., Chan, S., Wong, E., *et al.* (2006) The effect of problem-based learning on students' approaches to learning in the context of clinical nursing education. *Nurse Education Today*. **26**, 430–438.

Van Berkel, H.J.M. & Dolmans, D.H.J.M. (2006) The influence of tutoring competencies on problems, group functioning and student achievement in problem-based learning. *Medical Education*. **40**, 730–736.

Wood, D.F. (2003) ABC of learning and teaching in medicine: problem based learning. *British Medical Journal*. **326**, 328–330.

3: Readiness for problem-based learning

Juan Delport and Steven W. Whitcombe

Introduction

This chapter will consider the concept of 'readiness' as applied to problem-based learning (PBL). In doing so, we will propose that the educational assumptions underpinning PBL, and consequently, effective PBL opportunities, require both students and PBL facilitators to be ready for this particular method of learning. In our view, individuals' readiness for PBL is closely associated with their previous experiences of learning/teaching, coupled with their expectations of what is to be gained from a PBL programme. A mismatch between the espoused philosophy of a PBL programme and an individual's expectation and experience of learning may create the psychological phenomenon known as *cognitive dissonance*. Therefore, the exegesis of 'readiness' and its relationship to PBL require an examination of cognitive dissonance and its associated implications for PBL facilitators and students. We will further argue that cognitive dissonance theory provides a useful framework for understanding the positive and negative aspects of an individual's engagement with PBL.

Defining PBL

A simple definition of PBL is complicated by the issue that PBL, as a construct, has been used to describe heterogeneous educational practices (Maudsley, 1999). However, the basic principle behind PBL is learning that is initiated from the outset through the use of a problem, puzzle or case that needs to be solved (Duch *et al.*, 2001). Thus, PBL differs from other learning methods such as problem solving, by virtue of the fact that problem scenarios are used to drive students' learning from the very beginning of their course of study. Epistemologically, the practice of PBL challenges traditional (didactic) forms of learning through the process of problem resolution initially without access to foundational or propositional knowledge via, for example, lectures. This is because a primary goal of PBL since its inception (Chapter 2) is not the repetition of knowledge *per se*, but the contextualisation of knowledge to a particular problem.

The focus on knowledge contextualisation has made PBL a popular method of delivering professional programmes of study, for example, medicine, nursing, social work and the allied health professions. However, because of this focus, PBL makes demands on learners that are different than what may be required in traditional methods of teaching (Clouston & Whitcombe, 2005). Students need to be proactive in engaging with information that is relevant to a problem that exemplifies a curriculum area. PBL characteristically takes place in small peer groups in which a course tutor has a facilitative role. Through an interactive process, which most likely involves several iterative cycles of selecting information, processing and presenting it and then building on it following group discussion, feedback, reflection and critical thinking, knowledge and skills are gained. At its core, PBL requires a willingness to move beyond received knowledge into an active, self-directed process of challenging and testing knowledge to accommodate new ideas, associations and behavioural scripts that underpin the systematic development of meaningful professional roles and competencies. Rather than splitting theory and practice, PBL emphasises that this process of cognitive accommodation is facilitated in an applied context. This results in an internalised understanding, consisting of knowledge and skills, applicable to performing a professional activity safely and effectively in a given setting.

The concept of readiness

The notion of readiness stems from the work of Jean Piaget, an eminent developmental psychologist of the twentieth century. Piaget's (1953) observation of the intellectual development of children led him to describe complementary processes of incorporating knowledge into existing knowledge structures (assimilation) and of modifying the structures themselves (accommodation) in order to form a new understanding of the world. Contrary to the prevailing understanding, during Piaget's time, something more than rewards or punishments was required to foster learning new concepts – the child's mind had to be *ready* to do so. Effective teaching is more than conveying knowledge and information to passive recipients, but actively guiding a child's own discovery of the world.

Piaget (1975, 2000) pulled together a wealth of studies investigating the thinking of 4- to 12-year-olds in which a cyclical process he called *reflective abstraction* was described. Basically, this consists of a cyclical sequence: repeated actions introduce variations. The child notes both his or her actions and the effects produced. The child is able to differentiate and integrate new internalised objects. As a result of reflective abstraction, the child acquires new, co-ordinated actions. For example, in trying to press a soft ball to his or her mouth in order to suck it the way he or she would a breast or bottle, the ball may slip out of the child's grasp, drop and roll away. This produces sensations different from the familiar ones produced by sucking it. Should someone return the ball, a novel social response is also part of the new experience. Through repetition of these variations, the child notes his or her own actions, either grasping and sucking the ball, or releasing, dropping and possibly having it returned. This is the basis for reflective abstraction through which objects are differentiated; the ball is treated less as a breast or bottle and more as a new object. New experiences cannot merely be assimilated into existing cognitive structures; novel concepts are accommodated; increasingly complicated actions are co-ordinated: the ball can be grasped and brought towards the mouth or thrown away as a signal for social interaction different from that involved in feeding. This example illustrates the active nature of the learning process.

Readiness, andragogy and PBL

The educational principles underpinning the practice of PBL, notably problem resolution, co-operative learning, knowledge application and contextualisation, stem largely from the work of Malcolm Knowles and his views of how adults learn.

Knowles (1980) developed the theory of andragogy initially as a means of differentiating how adults learn from children. Whereas children's learning is largely directed by adults and motivated by extrinsic factors, for example, the desire to pass exams or please the teacher, adults, on the other hand, are self-directed and are generally more motivated to learn by internal factors such as increased self-esteem. In advancing his theory of andragogy, Knowles presents a number of assumptions concerning how adults learn. One of these key assumptions is adults' readiness to learn. For Knowles, 'adults are ready to learn those things they need to know to cope with their life situations or human needs' (Knowles et al., 2005, p. 61).

Knowles' concept of readiness differs from that of Piaget by means of a humanistic emphasis on the reasons for learning rather than the cognitive structuring (and restructuring) acquired through learning. However, both interpretations of what is meant by readiness are significant with respect to PBL. Piaget's (1955) view of the human mind developing through an ongoing process of creating and recreating maps of reality has an ontological resonance with how knowledge for the individual is utilised, applied and related to existing knowledge structures in the practice of PBL. Knowles' (1980) position requires us to ask questions such as how ready the individual is to learn in this particular way and whether, for example, the individual PBL student values learning through groups. Questions of how ready the individual is to accept the process of learning (e.g. knowledge contextualisation) and the approach to learning (e.g. group work, self-directed study) in PBL is pertinent to both students and staff on PBL curricula. What may impact upon their readiness for PBL is the dissonance encountered when faced with a new or different way of learning or teaching. Therefore, it is necessary to consider another psychological theory which is also pertinent to the concept of readiness, that is, cognitive dissonance.

Cognitive dissonance

Leon Festinger (1919–1989) created the theory of cognitive dissonance with the following simple assertions:

■ If a person holds two cognitions that are psychologically inconsistent or contradictory, he or she will experience an unpleasant psychological state called cognitive dissonance.
■ Because this state of dissonance is unpleasant, people find ways of reducing it.

It can be seen that Festinger's theory (1956, 1964) of cognitive dissonance combined cognition, what was happening in people's minds and motivation, and what this combination causes them to do as a result. This was a significant development on the social theories of the time, which was largely based on learning theory with its emphasis on observable behaviour. Cognitive dissonance challenged the long-standing dominance of reinforcement as an all-embracing explanation in social psychology.

Perhaps, the most famous dissonance experiment illustrating that human motivation cannot be accounted for by reinforcement alone involved the following scenario (Festinger & Carlsmith, 1959): College students performed monotonous, tedious tasks including packing, emptying and re-packing trays and turning rows of screws a quarter of a turn. They engaged in these repetitive activities for a full hour. After informing volunteers that this concluded their part in the experiment, the researcher then appealed to participants for help as a research assistant to stand in for someone who had not arrived. The researcher explained that he was investigating the effect of people's preconceptions on their performance of a task. An important research question was whether being told positive, negative or neutral things beforehand influenced the subsequent performance of the task. The next person who was about to participate in the study was to be told positive things. Therefore, participants were asked to tell the incoming research volunteer that they had just completed the task (which was true) and that they had found it interesting and thoroughly enjoyable (which was untrue from what they had just experienced). They were offered either $1 or $20 (which was quite a lot of money in 1959) to tell this lie. A key research question was whether being paid 20 times more to tell a lie would lead to people actually believing the lie they had told.

The results were interesting. Participants who were paid just $1 to say that they had enjoyed the boring task came to believe that it was actually true that they had enjoyed it to a far greater extent than those who had been paid $20 to tell this untruth. Reinforcement theory would have predicted that the magnitude of the reward should lead to people possibly accepting the statement. Dissonance theory made the opposite prediction. The knowledge that they had found the task boring was dissonant with the fact that they had told another person that it was enjoyable. To be paid a large sum of money to do so would reduce this dissonance by providing a situational incentive for telling the lie. However, if paid a small sum, $1, this external justification would be lacking, and the participant would feel the discomfort of the dissonance, and would, therefore, be motivated to reduce it. This they did by convincing themselves that the task was actually more interesting than it had seemed at first. By persuading themselves that the task had really been quite interesting, the magnitude of the lie they had told was reduced.

Another classic experiment illustrating that groups avoid dissonance and encourage conformity comes from the work of Schachter (1951) in which several groups of students discussed the case history of a non-conforming, rebellious, 'juvenile delinquent' called Johnny Rocco. After reading the case, each group was asked to discuss it and suggest corrective treatment, which ranged from 'very lenient' to 'very hard'. In these groups, consisting of about nine participants, there were three paid collaborators of the researcher. They took turns playing a role they had rehearsed beforehand; the 'modal' person went along with the group consensus; the 'deviate' took a position diametrically opposed to the group view; and the 'slider' started off in the deviate position and then shifted to the modal, conforming viewpoint. Schachter found that the modal person was the most popular one, showing the value placed on conforming to the group norm. The deviate was liked least. This finding has been replicated in a later study by Kruglanski and Webster (1991) who found that when a non-conforming viewpoint was expressed close to a deadline (when the group felt some pressure to reach closure such as needing to finish a meeting or reach a decision), the person expressing the dissenting opinion was rejected even more.

Aronson (1999a,b) points out that while conformity is important in some areas of life such as adhering to road safety regulations, there are times when conformity to group norms can lead to mistakes. Intelligent, confident people can change their opinions or behaviour as a result of real or imagined pressure from a person or group of people. This might be particularly intense during times when people are not sure about their initial positions or they feel the compulsion to be liked.

Aronson *et al.* (1991) designed an experimental situation in which students confronted their own risky sexual behaviour. This was based on the knowledge that while sexually active university students were in favour of using condoms to prevent AIDS and other sexually transmitted diseases, they simply were not using them. Therefore, Aronson and colleagues saw their task as creating dissonance between the person's positive view of themselves and the act of denial. To achieve this, they encouraged students to make a video, urging high school pupils to use condoms if they were sexually active. They were told that this video would be shown to high school audiences. In a comparison group, students simply reviewed the arguments for practising safe sex without making a video or taking on the role of giving advice to others. Both groups were then subjected to a 'mindfulness' intervention in which they were made mindful of the fact that they did not practice what they preached, so to speak. This involved asking participants to think about all those situations in which they themselves had found it difficult or impossible to use condoms in the recent past. In a comparison, no such mindfulness intervention was used. It was hypothesised that the highest degree of cognitive dissonance would be caused by the combination of making a video telling others what they should do to protect themselves and then also being invited to recall in detail all the times they themselves had failed to follow this good safety advice. The crux of the experiment was to see how the participants would reduce this dissonance, where it was predicted that the strength of their intention to use condoms in the future would be increased.

These predictions were supported. Furthermore, the higher dissonance group reported using condoms for a higher proportion of time than members of any of the other groups. These findings were reinforced when subsequently participants were offered condoms at a discounted rate. Eighty three percent of the high dissonance group took up this opportunity. Three months later, 92% of this high dissonance group were still using condoms regularly. These findings were significantly different than for the control conditions (Aronson, 1999b).

The hypocrisy-induction strategy discussed was also applied to other areas such as conservation of water (Aronson, 1999b).

Therefore, it can be seen that cognitive dissonance is a powerful construct that has been shown to generate significant attitude change that is not limited to trivial judgements about boring or contrived tasks.

Aronson's work particularly demonstrated that cognitive dissonance is especially relevant when a person's self-concept is threatened (Aronson, 1999b). Typically this happens when an individual behaves in a manner that is inconsistent with his or her sense of self.

Cognitive dissonance and PBL

Cognitive dissonance can be applied to PBL where the learner's or facilitator's self-concept is challenged by the educational approach of PBL. This could be because the approach is new or different from their previous experience of learning or teaching.

The application of cognitive dissonance to PBL will be demonstrated below through the use of two examples.

The first example cites how the experience of dissonance of some dental students on a PBL course impeded the process of accommodating new ways of learning. The second example highlights how dissonance was an instigator for positive change and active engagement in the PBL process for PBL facilitators on a nursing programme.

Shuler and Fincham's (2001) experience of delivering a PBL course for post-graduate dental students led them to identify how dissonance can be associated with group work in PBL. They argue that some dental students who started the PBL programme quickly became frustrated with the emphasis on group learning and sharing information, so much so that these students felt compelled to pursue all the learning objectives identified for a case (other than just their individual topics). This in turn caused conflict within the PBL group where others felt mistrusted by the participants who wanted to cover all the groups' learning needs themselves.

In trying to establish the reason why some students perceived the need to investigate the whole groups' learning needs, Shuler and Fincham discovered that, prior to starting the course, these students had been high academic achievers and had entered the post-graduate dental programme with good degrees from 'prominent' universities. Moreover, their previous experience of learning and resultant success had been largely dependent upon their individual motivation to succeed often in a competitive learning environment as opposed to the co-operative learning environment promoted through PBL. Thus, these academic high flyers felt reluctant to change a strategy of learning that had worked well for them in the past and, furthermore, did not wish to put their trust in other group members' research and knowledge, fearful that it may compromise their educational progress. As Shuler and Fincham (2001, p. 132) point out:

> The past traditional educational experiences of the students have a major impact on the transition to PBL pedagogy. Students who are 'super successful' in a high powered university must develop an incredible drive ... to achieve.

The second example of dissonance shows how initial apprehension and discomfort concerning PBL from the perspective of a facilitator can lead to shifts in teaching approaches and styles conducive to learning in a PBL environment. In a study of nursing tutors on a PBL programme, Wilkie (2004) explored the difficulties experienced by some tutors in matching the rhetoric with the reality of PBL. For the nurse tutors (facilitators) in Wilkie's research, adopting PBL as a teaching approach meant that they needed to promote a learning context that reflected a student-centred, process-orientated philosophy and a non-directive teaching style. However, for some tutors, particularly those anchored in a traditional view of education, which she termed the *directive-conventionalist* (Wilkie, 2004, p. 87), such an approach was challenging. The dilemma for these tutors and the cognitive dissonance that resulted arose from trying to select from an existing toolbox of skills, the ones that fitted most comfortably with the practice of PBL.

Wilkie's (2004) study was carried out over a 3-year period. Her findings revealed that in the first year, 'directive conventionalists' had problems relinquishing control of PBL groups. However, by the third year, many had become much more facilitative and supportive of students' learning. Wilkie argued that both through individual tutors' experimenting with PBL and by sharing their experiences, their approach shifted from information giving to information sharing. For Wilkie (2004), therefore, dissonance between existing teaching patterns and beliefs about PBL may be a catalyst for change. She argues further that the shift in approach appears to be less about the acceptance of a 'new belief system' and more about discovering how concepts of PBL can be utilised in practice. The caveat is, though, for a lasting and effective approach to PBL; facilitation tutors' behaviour needs to be compatible with their views and beliefs about the nature of learning. However, this study did reveal that the practice of PBL could prompt significant changes in approaches to facilitation in an attempt to counteract dissonance.

Conclusions

This chapter began with a discussion about the concept of 'readiness' and its relationship to PBL. We have argued that readiness for learning is a psychological construct which can be located in the work of the child developmental studies of Jean Piaget as well as the adult learning theories of Malcolm Knowles. Furthermore, we have suggested that to understand an individual's readiness for PBL, it may be helpful to consider the psychological phenomena of cognitive dissonance, which may be provoked in some learners and facilitators by PBL. Responses to dissonance are shaped so that cognitions are more consistent. In addition, this can be accompanied by attitude change and motivation to exhibit different behaviour. The resolution of cognitive dissonance aroused by PBL may facilitate or hinder engaging with it. Some dissonance-reducing responses, for instance, trivialising PBL, can block positive attitude change. The theory of cognitive dissonance has important implications for those wishing to facilitate and participate in constructive and effective PBL. It is worth emphasising the effort that will be required in forming cohesive PBL groups exploring a subject 'trigger'. PBL has been presented as a facilitative, learner-centred style for educating and training well-equipped health professionals for the challenges they will face in modern frontline practice. Students and staff can expect dissonance as part of this process. It can be seen as a way of experiencing tensions between what they know and do not yet know that might motivate them to minimise that state. PBL is intended to arouse this kind of dissonance, and then to channel behaviours that will reduce it in a productive way that fosters meaningful learning. However, any method of educating can be misused and can overlook the real needs of individual learners.

References

Aronson, E. (1999a) *The Social Animal*, 8th edn. Worth, New York, NY.

Aronson, E. (1999b) Dissonance, hypocrisy and the self-concept. In: *Cognitive Dissonance: Progress on a Pivotal Theory in Social Psychology* (eds E. Harmon-Jones & J. Mills), pp. 103–127. American Psychological Association, Washington, DC.

Aronson, E., Fried, C. & Stone, J. (1991) Overcoming denial and increasing intention to use condoms through the induction of hypocrisy. *American Journal of Public Health*. **81**, 1636–1638.

Clouston, T.J. & Whitcombe, S.W. (2005) An emerging person centred model for problem-based learning. *Journal of Further and Higher Education*. **29** (3), 265–275.

Duch, B.J., Groh, S.E. & Allen, D.E. (2001) Why problem-based learning? A case study of institutional change in undergraduate education. In: *The Power of Problem-Based Learning* (eds B.J. Duch, S.E. Groh & D.E. Allen), pp. 3–13. Stylus Publishers, Virginia Beach, VA.

Festinger, L. (1956) *A Theory of Cognitive Dissonance*. Tavistock, London.

Festinger, L. (1964) *Conflict, Decision and Dissonance*. Tavistock, London.

Festinger, L. & Carlsmith, J.M. (1959) Cognitive consequences of forced compliance. *Journal of Abnormal and Social Psychology*. **58**, 203–211.

Knowles, M.S. (1980) *The Adult Learner: A Neglected Species*. Gulf Publishing Company, London.

Knowles, M.S., Holton, E.F. & Swanson, A. (2005) *The Adult Learner*, 6th edn. Gulf Publishing Company, Houston, TX.

Kruglanski, A.W. & Webster, D.W. (1991) Group members' reaction to opinion deviates and conformists at varying degrees of proximity to decision deadline and environmental noise. *Journal of Personality and Social Psychology*. **61**, 212–225.

Maudsley, G. (1999) Do we all mean the same thing by "Problem-based Learning"? A review of the concepts and a formulation of the ground rules. *Academic Medicine.* **74** (2), 178–185.

Piaget, J. (1953) *The Origins of Intelligence in Children.* Routledge, London.

Piaget, J. (1955) *The Child's Construction of Reality.* Routlege, London.

Piaget, J. (1975) *The Development of Thought: The Equilibration of Cognitive Structures.* Basil Blackwell, Oxford.

Piaget, J. (2000) *Studies in Reflecting Abstraction.* Psychology Press, Hove.

Schachter, S. (1951) Deviation, rejection, and communication. *Journal of Abnormal and Social Psychology.* **46**, 190–207.

Shuler, C. & Fincham, A. (2001) To admit or not to admit? That is the question. In: *Problem-Based Learning – Case Studies, Experience & Practice* (eds P. Schwartz, S. Merin & G. Webb), pp. 126–134. Kogan Page, London.

Wilkie, K. (2004) Becoming facilitative: shifts in lecturers' approaches to facilitating problem-based learning. In: *Challenging Research in Problem-Based Learning* (eds M. Savin-Baden & K. Wilkie), pp. 81–92. The Society for Research into Higher Education & Open University Press, Maidenhead.

4: Developing problem-based learning curricula

Lyn Westcott, Alison Seymour and Sara Roberts

Introduction

The purpose of this chapter is to consider issues related to developing and delivering a problem-based learning (PBL) curriculum. Whilst the work that we share here comes from our experience of developing whole curricula at both undergraduate and postgraduate levels in health and social care education, it is hoped that this chapter will be of interest to an even wider readership. So, whether starting from scratch or planning to introduce PBL principles within an existing structure or programme, you may find this chapter of interest. You may also find this useful if you are a student studying a curriculum that uses PBL.

The chapter aims to

- explore some benefits of a PBL-style curriculum for all those involved;
- help identify some of the complexity of curriculum/programme design when working with PBL;
- highlight the use of PBL within the current climate of higher education;
- discuss when PBL may be incorporated into a curriculum;
- consider the resource and staffing implications for PBL, which includes professional programmes where students experience hands-on practice as well as academic study as part of the educational experience.

The ever-changing climate of higher education means that educationalists continually face new challenges, roles and responsibilities. These concern our students, our subject material and the institutions where we work. Our experience as tutors using PBL influences our engagement in this challenge, solving the problems put before us in a creative way and realising the potential of what can be achieved.

Benefits of a PBL curriculum

PBL has found an important role in the education of health and social care practitioners and other professionals. This is due to the benefits that are recognised from this style of educational experience (see also Chapter 2). The benefits are not only useful to students but are also relevant to qualified professional practice. They include the following:

▪ Developing independent autonomous thinking within a professional context – practitioners are required to become lifelong learners and this is inherent in this experience (see also Chapter 14).
▪ Accepting responsibility for being a motivated adult learner (Biggs & Tang, 2007). This means that students are aware of their active part in the learning process, setting goals for learning and negotiating with staff rather than being passively led through a training experience. This way, students develop a commitment to using their own time in directing learning as they would when they become qualified.
▪ Working in a culture where learners are encouraged to continually question, explore and evaluate themselves, their peers, the content and the staff; students are therefore able to develop into reflective practitioners (Schön, 1983).
▪ Coping with team working and resolving group dynamics with colleagues, for the purpose of getting on with any given task is sound preparation for practice within settings where interpersonal factors are part of the working culture (see also Chapter 6).
▪ Developing strong professional identity by considering professional issues and contexts throughout the learning and becoming confident in articulating these.
▪ Integrating and consolidating learning throughout the PBL experience. This means students are encouraged to understand complex relationships between topics, not just the sequential study of discrete subject areas, for example, the relationship between anatomical knowledge and functional disability rather than anatomy of a joint followed by pathology of a joint, then functional implications of that pathology. Learning is therefore not confined and can be flexible and applied to any individual context, reflecting the skills required in professional practice.
▪ Facilitating deep learning from the onset that reflects the skills required to engage in the lifelong learning agenda.

Additional benefits for staff also are important and include the following:

▪ Working in an environment which encourages students to become experts through questioning and debate – education becomes ever changing, enabling staff to enhance their own continuing professional development (CPD) and knowledge base that grows alongside the student experience.

■ Maintaining the interest of staff in the content of the programme as the educational experience changes from group to group. Even if the instigating material remains constant, each group is unique and so is their debate, as this reflects the wealth of their experiences and exploration.

■ Maintaining a sense of reality through the process of challenge and debate whilst enabling the learning of new concepts – just as patients/service users challenge staff professionalism in practice, students challenge the staff and their role in the educational setting.

The authors do, of course, acknowledge that PBL may suit some learners more than others, especially at the start of higher level study or when changing to this method of learning. It is our experience, however, that with the right level of preparation and support, most learners are able to adapt to PBL approaches and reap the benefits outlined earlier, even if they have no previous experience of learning in this way.

Curriculum design in a complex climate – where to begin?

To set the scene and explore different curriculum designs, it is necessary to consider the wider contexts that shape curriculum development, irrespective of the decision to use PBL (Figure 4.1). The curriculum should be easy to understand for institutions and others commissioning or formally approving the programme, as well as staff and students. The design therefore should be such that all stakeholders clearly understand what is offered and how that curriculum will be delivered.

A clear structure

Curriculum designs that use PBL should essentially aim to enable a PBL process to occur. When educating emergent professionals, they should also enable growth of professional thought and reasoning. The curriculum does this through an appropriate succession of trigger problems or issues to investigate, together with suitable structures for supporting learning that have been carefully planned at the curriculum development stage. Clarity in the structure therefore is crucial to guide the use of a PBL approach. Without a structure, the exploratory, emergent content agenda that seemingly flows when using PBL could be interpreted as boundary-free or even irrelevant to desired learning outcomes about professional skills and knowledge. This would be contradictory to the auditable, quality agenda that defines the higher education market in the United Kingdom. Learning in a PBL curriculum (like any other programme), cannot contravene the intended learning outcomes for a

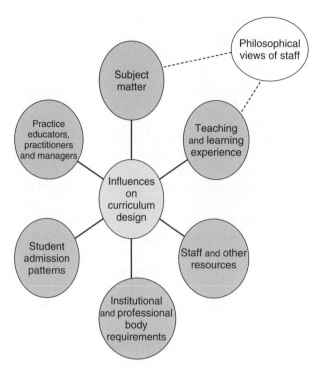

Figure 4.1   Influences on curriculum design.

particular profession or subject area. A clear robust curriculum design therefore can serve as an ally in quantifying a carefully chosen pathway towards the desired educational goal, as well as giving those involved in delivering the curriculum a universally understood framework for their work. The design should demonstrate to knowledgeable devotees of PBL, people with little understanding and even those who struggle to advocate its use, the validity of the learning enabled by the curriculum. The design should be able to demonstrate that the curriculum is fit for purpose and graduating students will be fit for academic award. It is useful to remember that any curriculum design must not only serve as a template for action but must also be a public window on the educational process that it offers – the robustness of PBL curricula in medicine and other health- or social care-related programmes being subject to public scrutiny through the UK media in recent years.

Factors that influence curriculum design

The design of any curriculum framework will impact on the teaching and learning strategy used irrespective of subject content. Design can vary from institution to institution, faculty to faculty and team to team. These curricula are influenced by a number of factors, some reflecting the philosophical aspirations of their creators and others the requirements of the wider context in which the curriculum operates. These are illustrated in Figure 4.1.

The value of ownership when changing to PBL

The drive for change to PBL may come from the institution, faculty or educational staff. It may emerge from reflection on student feedback or comment from the profession or practitioners. Whatever the drive, it is wise for curriculum designers to work hard in encouraging ownership amongst as wide a range of staff as possible in the process of designing a PBL (or indeed any) curriculum. Whilst democratic processes and group working in developing a curriculum can seem costly in staff time, this is a sound investment in the future delivery of the programme, especially one new to using PBL. Remember that PBL espouses the value of group learning; it makes sense then to draw on these benefits in curriculum design at either the initial conceptual level (when ideas are shaped onto paper), or even in the later operational stages (when the paper curriculum has to be put into action), a time when newer staff may come on board. Undoubtedly, a design that is 'owned' by the team responsible for delivering it will have vision and commitment from important stakeholders at the coalface, as well as providing a wider range of staff with project development experience. This will impact on the energy given to making the curriculum work well for all those involved, especially if PBL is new to key staff involved in its delivery. For professional programmes, it can also be wise to include a wider range of stakeholders in the development process such as practitioners who may be involved in future teaching or taking students for practice placement/work-based learning or service managers who will be the employers of future graduates. This involvement helps stakeholders in the profession understand the learning culture of graduates who have experienced PBL and be better prepared to assist their transition from university students to new health and social care practitioners.

Realism about constraints

It is important to realise that choices in constructing a curriculum design are constrained. Higher education courses in the United Kingdom and beyond are designed with particular exit awards in mind. These awards have to adhere to strict institutional (and often also profession specific) guidelines that govern level of study and the time commitment that students are expected to give. Subject matter may be clearly prescribed (especially on professionally driven courses), potentially contradicting the free spirit of investigation in learning that could be seen as the essence of PBL. Assessments are prescribed to gain access to exit awards, thus further constraining what is learnt and how this is demonstrated.

The influence of these constraints may still afford exciting opportunities for development in curriculum design but it is recognised that these circumstances will vary. Readers need therefore to consider their unique position and needs in developing any curriculum. It may be that an entire curriculum is not redesigned using PBL, for example, but planned as a component of a hybrid curriculum design sat alongside other teaching and learning techniques, maybe around a particular subject area or at a particular stage of the course. Such opportunities can be embraced, although designers should be mindful in enabling a meaningful fit with other elements that students will encounter in their studies before and after the PBL experience. This includes choosing appropriate assessments for PBL taught material that allow students opportunities to show fully their professional knowledge and expertise in a way that is sympathetic to this learning experience and the skills acquired because of it. This is preferable to using assessments more appropriate to a culture of traditional subject delivery with a narrow focus or scope.

Accommodating flexible study

Further complexity in curriculum design also comes from the commercial and flexible climate governing higher education policy and practice. Increasingly, UK institutions are changing traditions away from curricula only marketed to students that wish to see learning through from beginning to end in one place and on one particular course. The scenario of students 'carpet bagging' academic credit is very real. This can be from department to department towards programmes of integrated studies, or from institution to institution to upgrade awards like the UK foundation degrees to work towards a further professional qualification at a higher exit award. Whilst such initiatives widen access to higher education by enriching the expertise and experience mix in the student group, they present challenges to higher education staff. Those who effect decisions for Accredited Prior (Experiential) Learning (AP(E)L) schemes and those who are required to accept new students midway through a curriculum whilst releasing others to transfer elsewhere, need to be clear about learning achievements in their programme. They have to reflect carefully and quantify where in their programmes particular learning is achieved together with knowing which learning needs are still outstanding and where they are sited. In practice, this may be achieved through mapping learning outcomes for particular modules or linked to specific triggers or problems. This is extremely relevant now that there is a great emphasis on flexibility within universities in order to reduce the attrition rates and the consequential loss of revenue this entails. Designs have to be explicit enough to enable students to 'roll in and out' and succeed positively in their learning, irrespective of learning styles experienced elsewhere. Such shifts in study pattern expectations and provision thus reinforce the need for curriculum design to be flexible and adaptable to the climate of political and policy change. Whilst recognising that many students will be engaged in a curriculum from beginning to end, designers need to be transparent in their plan to allow these 'wandering learners' to engage flexibly in the learning and faculty administration needs of the PBL programme. Such thought will not only allow a fit and flexible curriculum to be put forward at any given time but will also encourage a resilient curriculum that is likely to endure the necessity for further change.

Learning with others

Similarly in professional education, as in health and social care, there is an increasing need to have a curriculum design that engages students in some form of inter-professional learning (IPL) or inter-professional education (IPE). Irrespective of the case for learning alongside student colleagues from other professions (this is discussed elsewhere in the literature), it is important to consider the type of educational experience that might guide and influence student expectations for inter-professional study. Students with a strong PBL experience may find themselves frustrated in a formal learning environment of, say, didactic lectures whilst students more used to a fairly traditional pedagogical approach may struggle if expected to function in an isolated module run using PBL. Such scenarios, unless well anticipated, could detract from the learning experience at hand. Careful consideration of learning needs, experiences and transparent negotiation with students about the style, practice and benefits of any given approach to IPL curriculum elements may help increase the benefits of this learning. It is also important to choose topic areas for inter-professional study with care. Using PBL within inter-professional student groups can provide an innovative and exciting opportunity for students to learn and develop together when an appropriate aspect of the curriculum is chosen. Exploration of multidisciplinary working, for example, would be an excellent aspect of the curriculum to explore together, whereas teaching a technical area like physiology, in isolation, without consideration of professional roles does not optimise the potential learning that might be gained from an inter-professional student group.

What are the curriculum design options that can accommodate PBL?

Curriculum frameworks can follow a number of overarching design types, which can overlap in practice.

- ▪ *Modular:* The learning is 'boxed' into discrete modules. Modules usually have an academic weighting, often in terms of a given level of learning that indicates the complexity of the material, and a corresponding time commitment attached to them. In the United Kingdom, modules generally follow a 1 credit = 10 hours study expectation, which includes contact time with staff and self- or peer-directed study. UK modules tend to have credits that are multiples of 5. This allows each module to have a particular focus and to sit flexibly within more than one curriculum if required. IPL is often linked to particular modules. Because modules generally need to be assessed independently to meet university regulation, students can compartmentalise their learning without making the necessary links to the content of other modules in a programme of study. This can be avoided by either having a series of modules that develop in complexity one to another (see spiral design below). Alternatively, concurrent modules can require application and synthesis of concepts covered elsewhere to guard against compartmentalisation.

■ *Linear:* The learning runs through a significant period of time (e.g. a semester or academic year) without being further subdivided. This allows themes to be linked and integrated within the learning that takes place, which is seemingly flexible and attractive to PBL. It may lack the structure to be transparent about content however, and mean it is more difficult for students to transfer in and out of the programme. This option is less preferred by UK universities.

■ *Spiral:* In a spiral curriculum, themes are introduced towards the beginning of a programme, then revisited with increasing complexity as the curriculum unfurls (Harden & Stamper, 1999). This type of design can be adopted within either a modular curriculum (say as an explicit themed strand of modules that run through the programme), or within a linear design, although good signposting would be required to help identify how these themes or topics re-occur.

■ *Subject specific:* Subject areas are clearly delineated and learnt together, say in particular modules. This is challenging to the ethos of PBL where problems are explored in a more integrated way but may be favoured as parts of hybrid curricula, especially for distinct areas like foundation sciences or research design.

■ *Integrated:* Here, a wide range of subjects are learnt together as relevant to a particular focus, say, by linking a professional problem or personal profile of someone seeking help from a professional service. This is a logical style of curriculum for PBL, recognising the synthesis of learning needed to understand and work with a given problem or scenario.

Irrespective of the design(s) chosen, it is important that each aspect of the curriculum content is planned carefully to relate well with the other components of the programme. Although problem-based learning can be accommodated in modular or linear programmes, for example, it is important that the learning is aimed to be progressive and developmental, moving from simple to more complex issues logically and with transparency. Each trigger/problem constitutes part of a wider whole that forms the entire curriculum. In this way, an accumulation of knowledge and understanding can be covered; this is especially useful to demonstrate in a profession-specific curriculum. This can be tracked through the progressive development of a variety of learning outcomes to guide the learning throughout the programme. For PBL curricula, learning outcomes need to reflect the essence of the PBL experience; they may require development of problem-solving skills or integrated understanding of a range of topics rather than narrower knowledge-based competencies. The overview of content shown in the curriculum documentation should be tightly and clearly 'constructively aligned' (Biggs & Tang, 2007), which means that the content proposed enables students to complete the learning outcomes set out for each curriculum element and not more than that, and the assessments should be based on allowing students to show they have achieved all of the learning outcomes. This aims to avoid duplication in the curriculum, although wider and deeper aspects of key areas can be developed in a spiral design with good effect. A developmental or sequential approach to content can be encouraged through involvement of a range of stakeholders in the curriculum design, especially as decisions are made on a suitable range of triggers/problems to structure the programme. Whilst many staff are primarily involved in discrete elements of any given curriculum, duplication in content can be prevented through staff awareness of the wider picture of how their element fits into the whole programme – this is easier when staff have been involved in the curriculum design process.

In addition to a developmental sequence of problems for the content focus of the curriculum, the design also needs to be clear about how it develops the thinking and skills of enquiry used by students. These are linked to the academic level of studies throughout the development of the programme and can be reflected in the wording and demands of the learning outcomes prescribed. Learning outcomes are often written with reference to educational standards documents, which delineate the expectations that can be reasonably expected at different levels of study, although educational teams need to ensure that the list of learning outcomes is realistic for the study-time allowed. In this way, students can be enabled and guided to develop their academic confidence as well as the skills to cope successfully with more complex situations as they progress towards completion of their studies.

To encourage students to meet the increasing demands within a curriculum, it is useful to devise guidelines for both students and staff that explain the expectations of PBL for any given level of the programme. In our experience, this is useful to enable people to meet the required standard of work whilst also helping to manage some of the uncertainty that can detract from the learning opportunities available on a PBL programme. Uncertainties among students can include whether they have worked to the expected depth of the task or if they have met the learning needs of themselves or the group. Guidelines may suggest ways to further assist working around the given trigger or problem, with strategies such as group or individual learning contracts, drawing on students' resources to guide and structure the learning experience with the guidance of a tutor (Whitcombe, 2001; Matheson, 2003).

Incorporating PBL into curriculum design

When considering introducing PBL into a curriculum, it is important for the planning team to think through when PBL may be most appropriate and effective and how this links to the overall style of the curriculum. As outlined earlier, PBL can be used as the overarching teaching and learning method for the whole programme or introduced in discrete stand-alone modules or elements of the curriculum.

At the curriculum planning stage, consideration should be given to the knowledge and skill level of students who will be studying on the programme, either in respect of the levels that they are likely to possess when they start the programme, or will need to develop as part of their new curriculum. This includes existing study skills and how to develop these appropriately for successful PBL, particularly if they have not previously experienced learning this way. It may be helpful to produce comprehensive study guidelines that clarify expectations of students and allocate time within the curriculum for students at the start of their PBL experience to develop the necessary skills to adapt their way of learning to suit PBL. Students should be fully aware of the demands of following a PBL curriculum before they commit to the programme or module, as some may need to make significant changes to how they learn and a level of honesty and commitment to this end will help make this process successful.

Although it could be said that PBL is an appropriate learning method for both undergraduate and postgraduate students who have been selected as being appropriate for this type of programme, our experience of working with postgraduate learners suggests that they are particularly able to utilise PBL effectively from the onset of their course. Perhaps, these students are quick to adapt to this method of study due to their maturity as autonomous learners. They enter with previous experience of study at a higher level and often have experience of the workplace, which seems to equip them with a range of skills that can readily be transferred into the PBL learning environment. Despite this experience, we would suggest that it is useful in the early foundation stages of any programme for postgraduate or undergraduate students to include learning opportunities that help students explore issues around group or team working and individual learning styles. This encourages students to think around issues linked to their own learning strengths and needs, which can then help students embrace the philosophy and commitment to self-directed learning that is so important in any curriculum utilising PBL.

Programmes that use PBL as the main teaching and learning method, we believe, face unique issues regarding student selection. In our experience, it is desirable, perhaps vital, to interview potential students as part of the selection process. Because of the responsibilities placed on students within a PBL curriculum, it is important that applicants know what they are signing up to and have an appreciation of what will be required of them as students. A useful selection process could involve finding out about students' understanding and knowledge of PBL, previous experience of group working and a simulated group exercise which could be observed against preset group-based criteria.

Undergraduate programmes that do not use PBL from the outset may find that PBL can be introduced in a staged or graded manner, either in modular form or working up to a fuller integration at higher levels of the course. As the curriculum develops, PBL may well offer an effective teaching and learning method for meeting more complex and self-directed learning outcomes. It is important, however, to prepare students for the change in expectations and responsibilities required if they are going to gain from this learning opportunity.

Any curriculum that incorporates PBL either as its main teaching and learning method or within selected elements, needs to consider what we call 'mid-curriculum blues', which can apply to both the students and the staff! This often occurs at the midpoint of a curriculum when initial enthusiasm starts to wane just when it may be difficult to see the end point of the programme. It can feel like being 'stuck in the mire' and relates closely to the theory of group processes and development (see Chapter 6). This can result in a reduction in motivation, creativity and commitment to the process of PBL. In order to avoid this, support and strategies need to be incorporated into the curriculum design, such as changing group membership, using a variety of triggers, timetabling in self-directed learning time and holidays. This is important, particularly when following spells of 'heavy' PBL commitments and using individual tutorial time with staff for added support and personal development reviews. It can also be useful to schedule in assessments at this midpoint of a curriculum rather than stack them up at the end of the programme. This can help students' motivation in terms of seeing progression and gaining feedback, which should be positive and constructive in order to support them through this sticky time. Being able to recognise and normalise 'mid-curriculum blues' is an important part of managing this process.

Implications for curriculum design – staffing and resources

When developing and delivering a PBL curriculum, the implications for staffing and resources need to be considered thoroughly at the planning stage to avoid difficulties later on. Good planning of resources needed for PBL along with an awareness of the implications for staffing should mean a better experience for both staff and students in the long run.

Implications for university staff

As previously discussed, staff involved in developing a PBL curriculum should be conversant with PBL as a teaching and learning method. Staff knowledge and experience needs to be considered in the planning stage. If staff have little or no previous knowledge of PBL, then careful consideration needs to be given to how they can develop the necessary skills and knowledge to plan and deliver the curriculum and support student learning via PBL. Resources for preparing staff for PBL should be tailored to meet individual needs, and adequate time should be given for staff to develop appropriately. Development should be cognisant of individual backgrounds and existing levels of knowledge and skills prior to the start of implementing a PBL curriculum. For example, staff who may have a great deal of experience of group-work in a clinical setting may need to adapt existing group-work skills from a clinical to educational setting, whereas an experienced lecturer of traditional lecture-based education may need to learn about the principles of group-work to feel prepared to undertake PBL teaching. It would be helpful if staff were able to chose from a range of different methods of learning about PBL, in particular the role of the PBL tutor – for example, the time being allocated to background reading, observing more experienced staff undertaking PBL tutorials or discussing and exploring PBL with experienced staff (it may be helpful to find other programmes, perhaps from different subject areas which utilise PBL to gather more diverse ideas). There also needs to be a plan in place to provide a good structure for supporting staff new to PBL once the programme has started. This could include peer review with other PBL tutors, reviewing audio-visual recordings of PBL group facilitation, discussion of personal reflections on group facilitation issues or seeking feedback from students.

It is particularly important when considering the different personalities that can make up a teaching team to consider including the practice of regular staff reviews of group progress to ensure consistency across the programme and to avoid giving mixed messages to students. Staff will often facilitate PBL in different ways; this should be considered to be a positive rather than a negative aspect of curriculum design as students will benefit from being challenged in different ways by tutors with different styles.

Staff teams also change over time and this should be considered within the planning stage to ensure that the overall curriculum is not adversely affected. Staff changes should be accommodated within the curriculum structure with new members of staff being given the opportunity to learn about PBL as outlined earlier.

Implications for professional practice

Within programmes leading to a professional qualification, there is often a requirement for students to undertake a period of study in a practice or clinical setting. This is more often than not a practice placement when students are assessed by a placement educator or mentor and have specific learning needs to be met within a particular timescale. Although the learning outcomes are normally specified as part of the overall curriculum from the university, the method of learning and the way the learning outcomes are met are often dictated by the field/clinical staff. When planning a PBL curriculum, this can raise a number of issues that should be considered by the university, the students and the clinical/placement education staff. It is vital in the curriculum planning stage that the potential pitfalls are acknowledged and addressed prior to students beginning their practice/clinical experience.

With this in mind, there are a number of issues that could be considered for students who use PBL as the whole or part of their learning at university. Perhaps the most important aspect to consider is the culture of the practice setting and the attitude of the placement educator. There are practical implications for practice educators accepting a PBL student onto a placement and there is a clear role for the university to support and facilitate the development of PBL knowledge and skills for all placement educators who plan to accept students into their practice areas.

PBL encourages students to investigate and challenge established ideas and be creative in how they solve problems, and this should be acknowledged when planning to take a student who utilises PBL on practice placement. The placement educator should be able to work in a way that facilitates individual learning in much the same way as a PBL tutor would facilitate group learning in a university setting. For some placement educators it would be helpful for there to be a shift in attitude away from the more traditional 'expert' practitioner role to a more equal relationship which encourages students to be able to express their opinions openly and make decisions jointly with the placement educator on the focus of learning within the time available to them. It has been our experience that a learning contract is a particularly useful tool to ensure that the relationship and the responsibility for learning are shared more equally. This is particularly relevant when considering that students come to practice placement settings with a range of previous experiences which have shaped their individual level of knowledge and skills. Naturally, as with the complexities of designing a university-based PBL curriculum (explored earlier in this chapter), it is important that there is also a structure present to guide and support the learning during practice placement. Some practice educators may find it particularly challenging to have some of their practices explored and analysed by students. However, rather than being seen as students criticising practitioners, it can be seen as a constructive way of helping practitioners keep abreast with innovation, clearly articulating evidence that guides practice or working in partnership with students to enhance their own CPD.

It could be said that health and social care settings can be restricted in what they are able to offer to service users by policy, legislative or cultural and historical aspects. PBL students are by their nature creative in how they approach issues or problems and will therefore sometimes find solutions that are perhaps not the norm in that practice/clinical setting. Practice educators often find that PBL students add substantially to their services by bringing in fresh ideas as they approach situations from a different perspective and may use knowledge in a more integrated manner than students who learn in other ways. However, in order for them to be able to do this, there needs to be a culture of acceptance that PBL students have learnt differently and therefore at times may behave differently from students from more traditional educational backgrounds. It is therefore vital that practitioners who accept students from a PBL programme on practice placements are fully aware of the different nature of PBL, and inclusion of practice educators in curriculum planning and selection of students for PBL programmes can be extremely useful in supporting this.

PBL students can also be an asset to the multidisciplinary team because of their preferred style of learning. For example, students may choose to work with a different professional as part of ongoing work linked to a client in order to integrate learning about others' professional role, rather than spending a nominated day shadowing another team member, which is often a traditional part of the practice placement experience.

Resource implications

When planning a PBL curriculum, careful consideration needs to be given to the resources that should be available to ensure the maximum effectiveness of the programme. In our experience, the following considerations should be made.

▪ Allocations of staff time for facilitation of PBL tutorials to ensure students are accessing the right material with accuracy and at the right depth.

- Preparation time for staff is also needed to prepare and evaluate trigger materials and staff/student PBL guidelines, and also to check over materials produced by students.
- Additional time may also need to be allocated to deal with any potential group dynamic issues in addition to the timetabled sessions.
- On a practical note, the number of rooms available must be planned for as well as student resources such as access to libraries, including journals, books, internet access.
- Students should also be encouraged to use a wide range of other resources that will enrich their learning experiences, for example, voluntary agencies, service users and practitioners/clinicians, equipment providers, specialist staff who can give advice, community facilities and so on. It is useful for rooms to be available for students to book in order for them to meet outside of timetabled PBL sessions as peer learning groups.
- Consideration also needs to be given to how the PBL tutorials will be timetabled – for example, how often do the groups meet, is there enough time between each scheduled session available for them to complete the work necessary, what is the purpose of each tutorial and how often will the staff be needed? Without careful planning of resources, the programme may have teething problems, which could have been otherwise avoided.

Conclusion

In conclusion, this chapter has explored the complexity of developing PBL curricula and has explored a range of practical aspects that should be considered at the planning stage of any programme. The relevance of PBL to health and social care education has been discussed. We hope that we have clearly shown the relevance of PBL to education for health and social care practitioners by establishing that the skills and knowledge that students gain from learning using PBL (for all or part of their education) is invaluable in professional practice. The relevance of PBL to staff, students and practice educators has been explored within the context of the current higher education climate along with the practicalities that should be considered when designing a PBL curriculum in the context of a number of different curriculum frameworks. The relevance of planning to incorporate PBL within an inter-professional agenda when designing the curriculum, as well as ensuring the involvement of a range of stakeholders at the curriculum planning stage should be useful for those intending to use PBL within a programme.

It has been our experience that PBL is an invaluable tool in the education of health and social care professions. This is because students who have learned via a well-planned PBL curriculum will find that they have been encouraged to develop professional skills from the start of their educational experience and a process that should continue throughout their professional lives. For this to happen, all those involved must be aware of the commitment that a PBL curriculum will demand, and this starts from the very beginning of planning the curriculum. Ensuring that all stakeholders involved have a vision of PBL from the planning stage onwards will ensure that the teaching and learning will be successful.

References

Biggs, J. & Tang, C. (2007) *Teaching for Quality Learning at University*, 3rd edn. The Society for Research into Higher Education and Open University Press, Berkshire.

Harden, R.M. & Stamper, N. (1999) What is a spiral curriculum? *Medical Teacher.* **121** (2), 143–144.

Matheson, R. (2003) Promoting the integration of theory and practice. *International Journal of Therapy and Rehabilitation.* **10**, 264–269.

Schön, D.A. (1983) *The Reflective Practitioner: How Professionals Think in Action*. Temple Smith, London.

Whitcombe, S.W. (2001) Using learning contracts in fieldwork education: the views of occupational therapy students and those responsible for their supervision. *British Journal of Occupational Therapy.* **11**, 552–558.

5: Becoming a problem-based learning facilitator

Gwilym Wyn Roberts

Introduction

This chapter will look at the fundamental aspects of problem-based learning (PBL) facilitation and the skills expected of the tutor/facilitator. In doing so, it explores the concept of facilitation and the wider facilitatory role and highlights certain elements in order to gain a better understanding of how to effectively facilitate PBL.

The past decade has seen a significant shift towards observing and evaluating facilitation in PBL. Useful publications include Savin-Baden and Wilkie (2000), Gilkison (2003), Haith-Cooper (2003) and Clouston (2005). Whilst there is literature outlining the role of students in PBL (Schmidt, 1993; Barrows, 1998; Savin-Baden, 2004; Clouston, 2007), little is written about tutors' lived experience of facilitating the approach. Research regarding the characteristics of behaviours required from the tutor for effective PBL facilitation is still relatively underdeveloped. This may well be because of the individual and subjective way in which each tutor perceives facilitation.

In addition, PBL facilitation demands strategic planning. It is the process wherein a group identifies its purpose and goals, develops a vision of itself and then defines a course of action to reach that desired future. Facilitators need to be trained to creatively identify existing strategic initiatives within the PBL process. Such individuals' intent should be to pose the right questions rather than to find the right answers. Facilitators should not be the experts in PBL group strategy so much as the facilitators of its development, and their purpose should be to foster a positive vision of the future and then to lead the search to find innovative solutions for a given problem.

What is PBL facilitation?

Facilitation is defined by Burrows (1997, p. 401) as

> a goal orientated dynamic process in which participants work together in an atmosphere of genuine mutual respect, in order to learn through critical reflection.

Dolmans *et al.* (2005) view facilitation as scaffolding student learning by stimulating discussion, providing stimulus for elaboration, encouraging the integration of knowledge and promoting interaction between students. This is achieved by asking searching questions, encouragement, seeking clarification and providing insights to enhance the application of student knowledge. Facilitation is person-centred and collaborative, a process of synthesis, of shared learning and a means of developing critical and creative thinking. However, because facilitation is dependent on the development of individual personal and professional skills, defining the actual role of the facilitator remains elusive and only vaguely specified (Haith-Cooper, 2000).

Facilitator's role

Historically, PBL literature has described the tutor's role as one of a passive observer who contributes to the group discussion to ensure clarity of information, and questions to gain a depth of understanding and to elicit deeper learning. The challenge is for tutors to ensure that they *facilitate* learning rather than teach, and *enable* students rather than control them. This may constitute a change in role for tutors who are more familiar with didactic teaching methods, a situation that many may find difficult to adjust to. Tutors who possess a tutor-centred conception of teaching through experience with a subject-based curriculum do appear to have some difficulty adapting to the requirement of a problem-based pedagogy. The literature does suggest that expert tutors are beneficial especially early in the presentation of the material (Whitfield & Xie, 2002), or where the experience is not well structured (Sadlo, 1997). However, the notion that expert tutors can be too directive for PBL groups has been called into question by studies showing that students do not perform better or even worse with non-experts (Schmidt, 1993). Most studies support the selection of experts for tutors (Whitfield & Xie, 2002), and many advocate that students have an expectation that tutors will share their specialist knowledge in particular, in health-care related disciplines.

Traditional teaching styles have a limited part to play in achieving the aims of a PBL curriculum, and for students to benefit most from PBL it is necessary for tutors to become experienced in facilitation (Johnson &

Tinning, 2001). This is not an easy task, but it is fundamental to effective PBL.

Becoming a PBL facilitator

The decision to become a PBL facilitator should not be taken lightly nor should expectations of the role be taken for granted. It is difficult for some individuals with a particular expert knowledge in a given area not to enter academia on the premise of wanting to share such expertise. PBL requires the tutor to function as a group facilitator rather than as a transmitter of information. Tutor preparation is fundamental to its success and it is questionable whether PBL facilitation skills can directly be taught, or whether the ability to facilitate is naturally inherent. Approaches to PBL pay due respect to the contributions of both tutor and student and result in a shared learning process (Johnson & Tinning, 2001). Maudsley (1999) argued that a specific staff development strategy is required to assist tutors in developing their skills in facilitation and Ho (2000) found some positive results from a teaching development programme that was specifically aimed at bringing about conceptual change.

The extent to which individual tutors will be required to change their pedagogic practice in order to become effective PBL facilitators will of course vary according to their professional background, current values, beliefs and attitudes concerning learning and teaching, especially within health-care education. Academics might assume that tutors' conceptions of teaching change with experience, usually from being more tutor centred and content orientated to being more student centred and learning orientated. There is, in fact, little evidence of this, which is surprising considering the current directives and commitment to personal and professional development. All health professionals, including those in education, have a commitment to continuing professional development as a way of improving their practice and most are capable of assuming responsibility for their own professional growth and development in order to become more effective facilitators.

Facilitator's attributes

A tutor's personal qualities and attributes have a strong influence on the development of effective facilitation. To enable learning and open discussion, tutors need to be creative, open, flexible, positive, approachable, enthusiastic, motivated and honest in group settings. Barrows and Tamblyn (1980) suggest that facilitators enable learning by challenging thinking, asking leading questions and raising issues that need to be considered by the whole group. Facilitators have to challenge information and working patterns in groups, but should do so in a way that encourages and motivates, rather than negates participation.

Rogers (1983) maintained that facilitators are real people and that being honest in forming genuine relationships in the learning situation was an important aspect of effective learning. He also argued that positive regard, without conditions of worth, enabled facilitation. From this, an effective facilitator is someone who feels able to be his or her own self, a person with fallibilities within the learning environment, who can be honest about his or her limitations and challenges. Rogers also suggested that students' learning is more effective when they receive high levels of understanding and caring. He also maintained that respect, genuineness and empathy with the student resulted in greater problem-solving, more verbal responses, more involvement, more eye contact, higher levels of cognition and greater creativity. In this way, one can argue that effective facilitation acknowledges and values the unique individual student in an appreciative way. It should be recognised, however, that the qualities and attributes for effective PBL facilitation need time to emerge as tutors develop their confidence, skills and competency in working with small groups.

Developing the facilitator's role

PBL involves the tutor in a collaborative learning relationship with students. The role of the tutor in this context demands the following:

- The ability to create a climate for student-centred learning
- The flexibility to cope with changing student agendas
- The capability of responding to individual student needs within a group situation
- The capacity to engage students in reflective dialogue and critical thinking

(Schön, 1987; Chenoweth, 2002)

The PBL facilitator needs to negotiate new understandings, utilise effective interpersonal skills and promote open discussion in small groups (Connolly & Donovan, 2002). To achieve this, facilitators may need to redefine their relationship with students and with programme content (Wheelan, 2005). This involves facilitators' releasing control of programme content and the learning process and forming a learning relationship with students, trusting them to accomplish specific programme outcomes. It is important to recognise, however, that facilitation is developmental in nature and starts with group regulation. This assists groups in moving from a reliance on tutor input to a position where shared guidance and ultimately self-regulation become the norm. Students are then able to guide themselves with little need for any tutor involvement.

Moving towards self-regulation requires a contractual partnership which demands particular expectations from both students and tutors. From a tutor's perspective, this may involve the following:

- Having an understanding of PBL as a philosophy and a clear synthesis of what is expected of them as tutor facilitators
- Being critical of the level of intervention required at different times in order to meet different agendas
- Having the wisdom to make decisions as to the level of the expert knowledge shared
- Developing an ability to apply the principles of PBL in the context of the curriculum
- Being open, flexible and creative with each situation
- Determining what the ground rules are, together with group expectations
- Developing the ability to project confidence and competence in what is understood by effective facilitation
- Enhancing creativity to promote student-centred and self-directed learning
- Having the confidence to support groups when the solving of the problem fails
- Having the wisdom to encourage a more positive and solution-focused process to PBL
- Pushing the boundaries of problem-solving to look at situations with an appreciative eye

Arguably, facilitators need to strive towards a style and skill base that promotes student satisfaction and meets individual and group needs and learning objectives whilst also balancing a commitment to maintaining the boundaries and outcomes created by respective regulatory and professional bodies, the organisation and the curriculum.

What makes a good PBL Facilitator?

A number of researchers have identified what constitutes 'good' and 'bad' PBL facilitation, amongst them Savin-Baden and Wilkie (2004) and Jamieson and Macpherson (2004). When comparing the view of 'expert' and 'non-expert' facilitators, Gilkison (2003) describes specific behaviours that constitute (good) facilitation. She identified three major categories of intervention:

1. Raising critical awareness by asking questions, rephrasing questions and prompting the students for definitions, explanations or more detail

2. Facilitating the group process, including re-focusing the discussion, guiding the students, attending to the group dynamics and summarising discussions to indicate closure of a topic
3. Directing learning, including imparting information and telling the students what or how much they should learn

In the context of good facilitation then, is there a single facilitator style to which one should aspire? Riley and Matheson (2004) suggest that there are a number of factors that influence the effectiveness of PBL facilitation. In addition to a familiarity with the philosophy of PBL and the curricula, tutors require a shared understanding of the intended outcomes and use of self in the tutor role. Jamieson and Macpherson's (2004) study of PBL facilitation illustrates the different interpretations that facilitators potentially put on their role. In contrast to Riley and Matheson's findings, one participant considered it 'bad' facilitation to include themselves within the PBL group even to the extent of suggesting sitting apart. It is argued here that facilitators need to use their experience to promote an effective 'learning environment' within the group. Success will be dependent on confidence in the process and understanding of what is important in promoting group and team working. Tutors open up opportunities for thinking when they can rephrase the problem and provide similar examples or different contexts to promote the flow of ideas. This cannot be achieved by 'sitting apart'.

Support and preparation

Developing a good facilitatory style clearly requires support and preparation. Tutors often report that their first experience of a PBL group is very daunting because there is no clear template, no uniform way to follow. Their desire often is to have some sort of guide on 'what to do' and 'what not to do'. In the absence of a guide, the potential is there for individuals to fall into a more traditional tutoring role which involves sharing information in a didactic fashion. But producing such a guide becomes difficult because of the subjective nature of PBL facilitation. It is fairly common for tutors new to PBL to be expected to 'just get on with it' with little or no support or training. However, some level of induction is necessary for all tutors. Support can manifest in many ways ranging from formal training sessions to shadowing and mentoring experiences. The implication of this is that tutors may require a more dedicated facilitator/mentor relationship in order to fully realise their potential.

Becoming an effective PBL facilitator requires organisational and peer support. Individual academics and organisations need to seriously consider developing support mechanisms in order to ensure that effectiveness. When higher education institutions recruit academic staff who are new to PBL facilitation, time must be given for them to truly understand both their role and the nature of PBL in order to develop confidence in their abilities. Tutors need to develop a clear ownership of the PBL curriculum and a shared understanding of the nature of tutor facilitation to be able to create opportunities that foster students' creative thinking. This places a responsibility on universities to provide opportunities for mentoring, coaching, supervision and continuing professional development to help staff acquire effective skills in facilitation. Such opportunities may help tutors to balance challenges with reinforcement, encourage questioning and provide a context from which students can generate ideas.

The facilitation process

Criticism of group facilitation in PBL is often aimed at the differences in tutor input. The difficulty here is that each individual tutor brings to the process his or her own particular style and skill set. I have already pointed out that individual personality traits have an impact. In addition, the facilitator's style or approach may also reflect his or her philosophical stance; thus there may always be elements of difference (Johnson & Tinning, 2001).

Facilitating group processes

If tutors are committed to PBL as a philosophy, effective group facilitation is essential so that the process promotes and optimises student learning. The extent to which a facilitator should lead or direct a group poses a challenge for tutors. This becomes apparent when groups experience difficulty; does the facilitator step in to rescue the group or not? Purists would argue that direct intervention in this sense contradicts the very essence of PBL and self-directed learning. Others believe that it should be the responsibility of the tutor to guide and direct groups at times of difficulty by actively stepping in to rescue them at a certain point. The tutor's approach to facilitation in such circumstances might well depend on the students' experience of PBL and on group dynamics.

Students may challenge facilitators, especially when they actively encourage self-directed learning by reducing guidance as the group progresses. However, when such anxieties surface some dysfunction associated with PBL may occur including increased stress, less focused discussion, criticism, apathy, lack of meaningful interaction, conflict, unequal sharing of workload and the domineering members being more controlling. When this occurs, the tutor may have to facilitate opportunities for the group processes and dynamics to be addressed, and at times a contract and a set of ground rules may have to be agreed on. However, the aim should be for students to define their learning needs and then explore with the tutor what the expectations are and how these can be met.

The extent to which the tutor intervenes and directs problem resolution remains debatable. Empowering all group members to reflect is one way in which the whole group can take responsibility to air difficulties and clashes that may have arisen. Reflective practice is common in all health-care professionals, and by adopting such an approach, the facilitators should grasp the opportunity to explore their own actions and develop a level of self-awareness and responsiveness to others that can enable proactive change. Similarly, peer review systems and support from other tutors can enhance our understanding of how we actually facilitate (Johnson & Tinning, 2001). If tutor facilitators understand and respect group processes and dynamics, input levels can be adapted to meet the groups' recognised needs.

Managing conflict

Every tutor knows how difficult it is to criticise students constructively. Facilitators must ask themselves what it was that made them criticise successfully. What did they do, through good preparation, choice of words, patience or what else? Following reflection, engaging in such an exercise allows the tutor to set the foundation for better feedback behaviours, realising the resources and positive experiences. This basic principle of appreciative and solution-focused work allows the tutor to find starting points for individuals and collective solutions by focusing on positive experiences instead of problems. It is often when students are unable to move forward that conflict within groups surfaces. In this instance, student groups will look to their tutor facilitator for help. Resolving group issues may indeed be a learning experience in itself for students who are looking for a right answer. Schwartz *et al.* (2001) suggested that the concept of PBL may not work where dysfunction exists within groups, or where support from tutors is challenged. In addition, from a facilitator's perspective, it can be difficult to decide how much to facilitate change in group dynamics and, indeed, whether the main responsibility lies with the facilitator or with the student participants. Haith-Cooper (2000, p. 270) contended that facilitators do have to intervene and that, 'by focussing on group interaction intervention levels will be individual to the group's needs'. Sadlo (1997) found that initial problems and conflict within PBL may be put down to the relationship between students and tutors and the anxieties around that.

An important element of PBL is to encourage groups to address the issues themselves in the first place, and to convey that tutor intervention should be seen as the last resort. Common sense would say, however, that it is better to prompt the group to deal with conflict at an early stage, rather than let it fester. The role of the tutor therefore would be to remind the group of their responsibilities and invite them to revisit the agreed contract or ground rules. Such interventions can enhance students' confidence and assertiveness in preparation for working with different personalities in modern day inter-professional teams.

The facilitator as a resource

In addition to facilitating group processes, tutors must effectively facilitate students' knowledge acquisition and application. In health-care education there is also a requirement to ensure that students gain a sufficient depth of knowledge and understanding in subjects relating to their future professional practice. This raises the question as to whether a facilitator should be a subject expert. Arguably, being a good PBL facilitator is more important than being an expert in a particular subject and some programmes deliberately utilise non-expert facilitators within the academic team. It is suggested here, however, that enough subject knowledge to understand the potential of the problem in hand is desirable. However, we must not undervalue the extent and richness of experience and expertise that some students may bring to the group. At times, it is helpful to realise that the facilitator could confidently place responsibility for expertise in the hands of the students, with the tutor being expert at facilitation, not necessarily the topic

Effective facilitation may include not only active participation but also the sharing of some knowledge and experience. As many tutor facilitators in health-care education come with experience in a particular clinical area, most are likely to bring with them a wealth and richness of expert knowledge. In turn, it is reasonable for us to expect students to want to maximise on such expert knowledge in order to add to learning and to develop skills. From a responsible, co-operative and participative perspective, being seen as a resource would seem acceptable for most tutors. However, from a tutor-centred versus student-centred perspective, this may cause conflict between the expert and the facilitatory role. This dichotomy has resulted in an ongoing debate between what Boud and Feletti (1997, p. 8) have termed 'facilitation and case expertise'. Engel (1997) suggests that expertise lies in facilitation not knowledge, while Barrows and Tamblyn (1980) contended that facilitators should be a resource as experts. The main point here is that maximising on expertise can inevitably inform knowledge and address errors in information. Others would argue that non-experts may facilitate well but can allow incorrect information to be assimilated and important points to be missed, thus disadvantaging some students.

Arguably, possessing expert knowledge can at times become problematic for PBL groups. Tutors with expert knowledge are more likely to direct and guide the group straight to a solution without exploring the problem fully. The content of knowledge thereby given should enable, not inhibit, the problem-solving process (Clouston, 2005).

Focusing on the problem

The level of guidance a tutor gives and the nature of the questioning are crucial for effective learning. A PBL facilitator is likely to question whether any of the group members disagree with a particular statement or aspects of the information shared. They are also more likely to challenge the students with questions that allow them to take a step back from the problem in order to explore different options. In this manner, tutors can encourage students to look beyond the problem and potentially see the issues presented with an 'appreciative eye', as this can facilitate a more creative and open process for learning. Engaging in a more positive and appreciative element of PBL encourages the development of a more solution-focused approach. Solution focus is based on the following principles:

- An emphasis on what is going well
- Utilisation of existing resources and processes
- A belief in the client/student as the expert
- Simplicity
- The inevitability of change
- A present and future orientation
- Cooperation
- Replication of existing successful strategies
- Replacement of unsuccessful strategies

(Mortesen, 2005; p. 110)

As such, facilitators who encourage a more solution-focused context in PBL may encourage students to be less concerned about how problems develop than in how they will be solved. Imagine a PBL session where all the students focus on forward-looking possibilities and not where things went wrong. Some may find this idea simplistic – nice and positive. According to McKergow and Clarke (2005, p. xii), 'simple is not simplistic; to be less simple, to take less direct routes involving a priori problem analysis, weakness diagnosis and any of the myriad potential excursions and pitfalls, is to risk at best expending more resources and time than necessary, and at worst spreading confusion and making any problems significantly worse'. Allowing students to become too focused on problem-solving may give them the wrong perception of PBL. If the use of PBL in health-care education is to develop competent practitioners who are lifelong learners, then allowing students to over-focus on the problem may become a false reality. When considering therapeutic intervention in health-care practice, client's problems may at times be unsolvable for a variety of reasons. All health-care practitioners can aim for is to facilitate a process by which clients adapt to living with their disability or illness. Similarly, it is important for the tutor to facilitate students to explore options within this scenario. If problems presented within PBL are seen by students as unsolvable, they may be unable to move forward or believe that they are not functioning well. In addition, when a student's contribution to the group is deemed to be incorrect or a group is heading in the wrong direction as far as their learning is concerned, then the tutors' intervention must be timely.

The role of the tutor in this sense is to put aside expert knowledge and offer reassurance by allowing students to retrace their path to see whether any alternative routes or even mistakes can be identified. In addition, the tutor may encourage students to approach the problem from a different angle, with an appreciative eye first (see Chapter 12). It is a tutor's ability to promote open appreciative thinking and visualisation of practice, through the use of imaginative trigger material that appears to have the most impact on students being able to think outside the box.

Creativity and PBL facilitation

Creativity requires tutors and students to work in novel and original ways that are appropriate to their work and circumstances. Enhancing creativity through PBL is the focus of Chapter 10, but to develop creative thinking it is crucial that the facilitator is not so much concerned with testing the students' factual knowledge as ensuring that they think about what they are saying, synthesise the material and adhere to the PBL process. The tutors' task is to engage students in the process, keep activities dynamic and creative, probe students' knowledge through questioning, modulate the challenge of the given problem and monitor the educational progress of each individual in the group. Arguably, tutors who have ownership of the specific curriculum and a commitment to self-directed learning are better placed to facilitate groups in a way that enables shared guidance and promotes creative thinking.

Riley and Matheson's (2004) study highlights the need for tutors to be more active in their role as facilitators and provides an ideational context for the problem to enhance students' creative thinking, develop ideas and promote further questioning. Constantly throwing questions back at students in a belief that this is effective PBL facilitation can inhibit the development of creative thinking and questioning. This passive style of facilitation can be viewed as 'opting out'. When this occurs, tutors may experience criticism from within the student group. Where direction is completely lacking and students feel pressured by constant questioning they often fall into the trap of believing that they are being tested or examined and may begin to disengage from PBL, and their learning becomes assessment driven.

How to give feedback

How students receive and embrace constructive feedback and summing up within a group process are two factors likely to influence and enable facilitation. The manner in which positive and constructive feedback is given to students is crucial to their personal and professional development within PBL. Feedback usually takes the form of highlighting positive contributions and challenges to content, knowledge and group process and dynamics. Facilitators can provide the opportunity for students to summarise and present key issues and explain and discuss them with others. They can also enable students to discover and explore personal meaning and develop tools for lifelong learning and, to evaluate feedback, reflect on their own learning to see how they are progressing toward meeting their learning objectives (Clouston, 2005).

Feedback from students

In PBL, feedback should be a two-way process. Therefore, feedback and evaluation from students may offer tutors some interesting and constructive pointers when considering effective facilitation. Using students' evaluation as part of feedback is central to any quality assurance mechanism. It is crucial that students' voices are heard as part of plenary and staff student forums. When receiving feedback from students, tutors need to acknowledge the often diverse nature of a student group based on gender, age, prior experience and how this might influence its uniformity and quality. In addition, the tutor may adopt the following approach to receiving feedback:

▪ Listen calmly to the suggestions of students and colleagues.
▪ Attempt not to comment on the feedback, nor defend the procedure.
▪ Thank the feedback givers and choose the suggestions which are useful to take away.
▪ Leave everything else behind.

A structured procedure may prove to be successful in giving feedback, and the following suggestions may be followed:

▪ (Students) – 'This is what we liked in the situation' (just praise, no hidden suggestions).
▪ (Tutor) – 'This is what I liked in the situation'.
▪ (Both students and tutor) – 'We will do this in the real situation again and we will try to do this differently next time'.

According to all experience, this sequence leads to feedback that is appreciative and which is accepted effectively. Mature students who have experience with small group work might have some constructive feedback to give based on past experience of what they think the tutor's attributes should be. Younger, less experienced students, on the other hand, may need encouragement and prompting to contribute, and tutors should see this as a particular aspect of their skills base. Asking encouraging or provocative questions may prompt feedback. Alternatively, the facilitator may need to allow for confidence to build, without interjecting.

Evaluating the facilitator role

The skill of facilitating a deep learning experience and allowing students' knowledge, evidence and arguments to be self-directed pushes the boundary of what one might assume the role of the tutor to be. There are a number of ways in which students in particular can identify criteria for good facilitation. One way is to examine the existing evidence base around the role of the facilitator. Another way would be for students to directly observe facilitation in action and evaluate whether specific behaviours/interventions are consistent with the broad definition of the role of facilitator. To this end, some PBL programmes involve students in recruitment and selection processes for new academic staff, usually observing applicants facilitating a mock session as part of the interview.

In this way, observers can evaluate and question whether the 'would be' tutors focused on the process, were they inclusive and ensured that all students participated, did they probe and challenge the students' knowledge appropriately, were they too directive, did they use their expert knowledge and did they respond to the specific situation by probing further or suggesting a narrower focus, as required. In such situations, effective facilitation would be judged against the level of intervention and whether they guided students through the enquiry and decision-making process well and whether they challenged their assumptions.

Final thoughts

The role of the facilitator in PBL is both exciting and complex. Student, peer and organisational expectations are great and basic strategies and techniques can arguably be learned and developed to meet perceived needs. Tutors' recognition of their own personality, past experience and skill set, and including them all in the work environment are central to effective facilitation. Intrinsically, facilitation is inherently linked to who one is, and recognising the importance of personal differences enables a more balanced approach to tutor activity within PBL groups.

PBL presupposes a student-centred and learning-orientated conception of teaching on the part of the tutor. However, we have to recognise that tutors who have a tutor-centred approach through experience with a subject-based curriculum may well have some difficulty adapting to PBL. The level of involvement and participation within the group, including giving direction, guidance, support and sharing knowledge is integral to both group function and individual satisfaction. Generally, active participation in the group enables and empowers students to effectively learn, while a more reserved role may inhibit interaction and therefore be seen as purely observational and unequal in commitment.

Some level of support, flexibility, preparation and practice is integral to effective facilitation, and organisations need to seriously consider mechanisms such as formal training, mentoring and supervision to support tutors. In theory, continuing professional development and lifelong learning can offer opportunities to enable facilitators to become more effective and their practice to be evidence based, critically responsive to meet perceived needs of themselves, their students, organisations, professions and even the community of PBL practitioners worldwide.

References

Barrows, H.S. (1998) The essentials of problem-based learning. *Journal of Dental Education.* **62** (9), 630–633.

Barrows, H.S. & Tamblyn, R.M. (1980) *Problem-Based Learning, an Approach to Medical Education.* Springer Publishing Company, New York.

Boud, D. & Feletti, G. (1997) Introduction. In: *The Challenge of Problem-Based Learning,* 2nd edn. (eds D. Boud & G. Felleti), pp. 1–14. Kogan Page, London.

Burrows, D.E. (1997) Facilitation: a concept analysis. *Journal of Advanced Nursing.* **25**, 396–404.

Chenoweth, D.H. (2002) *Evaluating Worksite Health Promotion.* Human Kinetics Publishers, Champaign.

Clouston, T.J. (2005) Facilitating tutorials in PBL: a student's perspective. In: *Enhancing Teaching in Higher Education – New Approaches to Improving Student Learning* (eds P. Hartley, A. Woods & M. Pill), pp. 54–64. Routledge, London.

Clouston, T.J. (2007) Exploring methods of analysis talk in problem based learning tutorials. *Journal of Further and Higher Education.* **29** (93), 265–275.

Connolly, D. & Donovan, M. (2002) Introducing a PBL model in an occupational therapy course. *Learning in Health and Social Care.* **1** (3), 150–157.

Dolmans, D.H., De Grave, W.S., Wolfhagen, I.H.A.P. & van der Vleuten, C.P. (2005) Problem-based learning: future challenges for educational practice and research. *Medical Education.* **39**, 732–741.

Engel, C.E. (1997) Not just a method but a way of learning. In: *The Challenge of Problem Based Learning,* 2nd edn. (eds D. Boud & G. Feletti), pp. 17–27. Kogan Page, London.

Gilkison, A. (2003) Techniques used by 'expert' and 'non-expert' tutors to facilitate problem-based learning tutorials in an undergraduate medical curriculum. *Medical Education.* **37**, 6–14.

Haith-Cooper, M. (2000) Problem-based learning within health professional education. What is the role of the lecturer? *Nurse Education Today.* **20**, 267–272.

Haith-Cooper, M. (2003) An exploration of tutors' experiences of facilitating problem-based learning. Part 2 – Implications for the facilitation of problem-based learning. *Nurse Education Today.* **23** (1), 65–75.

Ho, A.S.P. (2000) A conceptual change approach to staff development: a model for programme design. *International Journal for Academic Development.* **5** (5), 30–41.

Jamieson, G. & Macpherson, K. (2004) What makes a good facilitator. Conference on Problem Based Learning: A Quality Experience Across the Boundaries, Across the Disciplines and Across the Globe. http://www.usir.salford.ac.uk. Accessed on 30th April 2006.

Johnson, A.K. & Tinning, R.S. (2001) Meeting the challenge of problem-based learning: developing the facilitators. *Nurse Education Today.* **21**, 161–169.

Maudsley, G. (1999) Roles and responsibilities of the problem-based learning tutor in the undergraduate medical curriculum. *British Medical Journal.* **318**, 657–661.

McKergow, M. & Clarke, J. (2005) *Positive Approaches to Change: Applications of Solutions Focus and Appreciative Inquiry at Work.* Solutions Books, Cheltenham.

Mortesen, J. (2005) Solution focused strategic planning. In: *Positive Approaches to Change: Applications of Solutions Focus and Appreciative Inquiry at Work* (eds M. McKergow & J. Clarke). Solutions Books, Cheltenham.

Riley, J. & Matheson, R. (2004) The enhancement of creativity through problem based learning. In: *Higher Education Academy Imaginative Curriculum Workshop: Creativity Taught and Caught.* University of Strathclyde, Glasgow.

Rogers, C. (1983) *Freedom to Learn in the 80s.* Charles Merrill Publishing Co, Ohio.

Sadlo, G. (1997) Problem-based learning enhances the educational experiences of occupational therapy students. *Education for Health.* **10**, 101–114.

Savin-Baden, M. (2004) Problem-based learning: reason in madness?. Conference on Problem-Based Learning: A Quality Experience Across Boundaries, Across Disciplines and Across the Globe. Available at: http:www.//usir.salford.ac.uk. Accessed on 22nd April 2005.

Savin-Baden, M. & Wilkie, K. (2000) Understanding and utilising PBL strategically in higher education. 8th Improving Student Learning Symposium: Improving Student Learning Strategically. UMIST, Manchester.

Savin-Baden, M. & Wilkie, K. (2004) *Challenging Research in Problem-Based Learning.* SRHE & Open University Press, Berkshire.

Schmidt, H.G. (1993) Foundations of problem-based learning: some explanatory notes. *Medical Education.* **27**, 422–432.

Schön, D. (1987) *Educating the Reflective Practitioner. Towards a New Design for Teaching and Learning in the Professions.* Jossey-Bass, San Francisco.

Schwartz, P., Mennin, S. & Webb, G. (2001) *Problem-Based Learning, Case Studies, Experience and Practice: Case Studies of Teaching in Higher Education.* Kogan Page, London.

Wheelan, S.A. (2005) *Group Processes: A Developmental Perspective*, 2nd edn. Allyn and Bacon, London.

Whitfield, C.F. & Xie, S.X. (2002) Correlation of problem-based learning facilitators' scores with student performance on written exams. *Advanced Health Science in Education, Theory and Practice.* **7** (1), 41–51.

6: Managing group dynamics and developing team working in problem-based learning

Alison Seymour

Introduction

Working as part of a group is an aspect of problem-based learning (PBL) which requires the individual to be able to achieve task performance whilst also negotiating and managing group dynamics and processes successfully. This chapter aims to explore common aspects of group development and group dynamics which can manifest in PBL groups and explores how these processes can be understood and managed from both a student and a facilitator perspective.

The chapter also discusses how the skills that are required to manage group dynamics within PBL groups link to the development of transferable team-working skills, which are necessary for graduates both in health and social care settings and other professions.

Defining groups and teams

Levi (2007) suggests that groups are more than just a collection of people; they have characteristics such as a reason for existence, shared goals, a sense of membership and roles and rules that influence and control the interactions of group members. The distinction between groups and teams is often blurred. Teams can be seen to be a special type of group and the term *team* is most often used when referring to work settings. Work-focused teams are often characterised by their structure, defined goals and accountability for a common project. So how do PBL groups fit into these definitions? PBL groups are characterised by a collection of individuals coming together to work on a defined learning task. They have a shared sense of ownership and responsibility both to the task and to the group, and the members need to work cooperatively and in a self-directed way in order to meet each others' learning needs. This involves being able to focus on the task in hand whilst also managing the group dynamics and processes in a professional, constructive way. Hayes (1997), cited in Levi (2007), suggests that for a group to become a team, it must be empowered and have some authority to act on its own; this is an important aspect of PBL groups where self-direction is necessary for the achievement of their goals. It could be suggested that the process of working within PBL groups helps develop more specific team-working skills that can be transferred into professional practice. Due to the blurring of definitions in the literature, the terms *groups and teams* will be used interchangeably for the purposes of this chapter.

What are group dynamics and group processes?

The terms *group dynamics and group processes* are more synonymous with group psychotherapy terminology; however, the terms have relevance within PBL groups and other types of teams as well. Levi (2007) refers to group dynamics as the process of understanding how groups operate. Finlay (1993) describes group dynamics as being the study of the processes concerning the nature of groups and how they develop and work. She recognises that each group is unique and evolves in a different way depending on the individual members and the events that occur in the group itself. The term *group dynamics* tends to refer to the individual interactions between group members, whereas group processes are more concerned with the evolution or development of the group. Simply speaking, these terms are usually used to distinguish between the product, task aspect of the group and everything else that goes on within the group.

Group development

Finlay (1993, p. 66) suggests that 'groups that come together regularly over a period of time change and develop', but are the phases that groups go through predictable? Research into this question has been going on for many years and there are numerous models of group development within the literature. Wheelan (2005) provides a summary of these models which can be categorised as follows: sequential models (of which Tuckman and Jenson (1977) is one of the most widely known), cyclic models, life cycle models, equilibrium models and adaptive/non-sequential models. What is evident from these theories is that groups do develop and there are phases that can be recognised and predicted, which follow recurrent themes; however, the processes that groups go through depend on the context and circumstances of the group. It is useful for PBL group members and facilitators to have an understanding of these processes in order to maximise functioning within PBL groups.

Wheelan (2005) proposes a developmental model of group development, essentially a life cycle model, which is informed by and integrates
aspects of other group development models. It is a five-stage process
that resonates closely with pertinent aspects of PBL groups.

■ **Stage 1: Dependency and inclusion**. This initial stage is characterised
by dependency on the group leader who will usually be the group
facilitator at the beginning of a PBL group. The leader is seen as benev-
olent and competent and is rarely challenged. They are expected to
provide group members with direction and personal safety within the
group. Group members are concerned with acceptance and inclusion
in the group and communicate in a tentative and polite way with each
other. There is often a lack of group structure and organisation and
the formation of subgroups is rare at this stage. The goal of this stage
is to create a sense of belonging and establish predictable patterns
of interaction which help create a sense of safety and loyalty to the
group. Once this is established, the group members are able to begin
to contribute to accomplishing the group task.

■ **Stage 2: Counter-dependency and fight**. This stage is characterised by
conflict either between group members or with the leader. The leader
may be challenged and disagreements about goals and tasks emerge.
Because members feel safer, they are more able to dissent and deviate
from the emerging group norms. Members lose their dependency
on the leader and there is less conformity. It is important for group
members and facilitators to remember that conflict is not necessarily
destructive to the PBL group; in fact, if management and resolution
can be made, then increased trust and cohesion can be developed,
which helps the group move into the third developmental stage.

■ **Stage 3: Trust and structure**. At this stage trust and security will
emerge in the group, more mature negotiation of group goals, organisation and roles are evident and communication becomes more open,
flexible and task orientated. Although conflict may still be present,
it is less intense and members are able to utilise conflict resolution
strategies more effectively. Peer feedback is possible and tends to
be more related to the task and information is shared rather than
used as a way of gaining power and status within the group. This
stage indicates that the group is preparing to work and commitment
to individual and group goals is strong. Group cohesion, trust and
member satisfaction increase.

■ **Stage 4: Work**. This is the optimum working stage of the group. In
PBL groups, it can be observed that members are focused on getting
the job done well and maintaining a high performance for a period
of time. Group members remain cohesive whilst focusing on the task
effectively in order to produce a high standard of task performance.
Roles are accepted and used to promote high performance and

quality and the leadership style emerges to match the group's needs. The group is able to tolerate subgroups and member deviance, and member attraction and cooperation is high. During this stage, group members are able to seek out and optimise the resources available to them and match individual expertise and materials to accomplish the task successfully.

▪ **Stage 5: Termination**. Group endings and changes in member make-up differ within different PBL curricula but it is inevitable that at some point groups will terminate and the membership will change. This is actually a useful thing to occur throughout any PBL programme as groups that work together for too long can lose creativity and motivation. Impending termination of a group, however, can result in a group regressing to earlier stages and it is useful for members to be able to discuss this and prepare for termination. Groups may react in increased solidarity and are able to discuss achievements but similarly stress and anxiety may be evident, with avoidance of dealing with problematic issues. It can be useful for the group facilitator to make the group aware of these processes in order to facilitate a positive end for the group. This can be achieved through individual and group reflections.

This developmental model of group processes, perhaps, suggests that all groups go through these stages. This is not necessarily so and groups, like people, can get stuck at any stage or regress to previous stages depending on the circumstances. These may include significant changes in group membership, external demands of individuals, psychological changes in group members and serious internal conflict. Students and facilitators exist outside of the PBL group and their individual needs and circumstances can have a significant effect on group processes. What appears to be important is that both members and facilitators have an understanding, are aware of group development and are able to reflect on and discuss how the group is functioning at regular intervals.

Managing group dynamics and processes: common challenges and solutions for PBL groups

Working as part of a PBL group can initially be daunting for both students and new facilitators. On the surface, it may look like an informal, relaxed and learning environment but very quickly it becomes evident that a high level of communication skills and self-awareness are required to pick your way through the subtlety of what is required in order to achieve both task performance and constructive group functioning. The following section summarises the group dynamics and processes that students and facilitators often find the most challenging in PBL groups. References to unpublished observations and quotes are taken from my research undertaken with post-graduate students on their experiences of managing group dynamics in PBL groups.

Individual personality issues

Feedback from student group members indicates that two polarities of personality types cause the most tension within PBL groups (unpublished observations). These are the dominating and the silent members, and such observations are well supported in the literature (Finlay, 1993; Corey & Corey, 1997; Yalom & Leszcz, 2005).

The dominating group member

Yalom and Leszcz (2005, p. 391) refer to this member as *the habitual monopolist* and he or she tends to be evident and most problematical in the early stages of group formation. Group members often think that in order to be a 'good' group member, it is necessary to say a lot and the monopolist will quickly fill this role. Contributions are often related to one's own self and the monopolist will pick up on other members' comments and personalise these, relaying anecdotal and often irrelevant stories. Initially both facilitators and members find this role useful as it means that they do not have to say anything and can be relieved that someone else is doing all the talking! However, this can quickly lead to irritation and resentment in the group and become a source of conflict. This behaviour is often a result of lack of confidence in the individual or could be due to his or her trying to establish themselves in the group or attempting to take control. If you have several dominating members in a group who are allowed to monopolise early on, the group can quickly lose motivation and this prevents group cohesion developing. It is very important that the monopolist is dealt with in a sensitive way and it is often a role which initially should be taken by the group leader as during the first stage of the group members will be looking to the leader to guide and support them. It is natural for group leaders to want to close the monopoliser down as the affects on the group as a whole become evident. This needs to be done in a supportive way so that the monopoliser does not feel picked on or scapegoated by the leader as will be closely observed by the other group members who need to feel that the leader is not only in control, but is also working for the good of all the group members. There are several techniques that can be used.

▪ Sitting next to the monopoliser (Finlay, 1993). This technique reduces eye contact between the leader and the group member and, therefore, reduces encourager-type non-verbal communication. Monopolisers will often look to the leader for feedback and reassurance and this can be kept to a minimum if eye contact is reduced.

- Allowing the monopoliser space to talk but interjecting and asking for other group members' opinions.
- Encouraging them to say more by asking focused questions about the topic in discussion rather than letting them dominate with anecdotal story-telling.
- Placing the responsibility back on the group and asking the group if they are happy with allowing the individual to carry all the responsibility for talking! This is often best done in a humorous way to avoid the group feeling that they are being 'told off' or humiliating the monopoliser.

Developing group guidelines at the beginning of the PBL group can be a useful way of avoiding this problem getting out of hand in the first place (Baptiste, 2003). Encouraging guidelines which value individual contributions and explicitly outline that all group members are expected to contribute to discussion gives a vehicle for the leader and members to revisit if this is not occurring within the group. A further technique which was used by a group, where it was openly acknowledged that monopolisers were at work, was the use of a talking stick. The rule in this situation was that you could only speak if holding the stick. The group found this a useful, light hearted way of challenging the dominant personalities in a constructive way. Occasionally, it is necessary for the facilitator to speak to an individual outside of the group but it is much more powerful if this problem can be managed within the group by the group members.

The quiet or silent member

This type of behaviour can cause as much frustration and tension for group members and the facilitator as the monopolist. There are many reasons why a member may be silent within a group (Corey & Corey, 1999; Yalom & Leszcz, 2005) but the silent member is often perceived by other group members as withholding, not engaged in the process or bored. Whatever the reasons, this style of behaviour can have a damaging effect on the development of the group process and internal dynamics. Again, in the early stages of a PBL group it is often useful for the facilitator to model ways of managing silent members and many of the techniques described above can be utilised as a way of encouraging increased participation. It is important to avoid consistently challenging a silent member in a group as this can lead to further withdrawal. Supportive encouragement of contributions by quieter members can help them to develop confidence and trust that the group is a safe environment in which to participate. Quiet members are sometimes useful members to utilise in specific roles within a group and it can be helpful to assign roles such as a group recorder or observer.

The recorder is responsible for keeping a record of the group discussion and feeding back decision-making and allocation of research, whereas the observer is assigned the role of reflecting on the group process and dynamics and feeding back to the group progress of the group. A word of caution is needed, however, as the quiet member may latch onto the role and hide behind it using it a reason to contribute less in the group discussions. One of the most effective role allocations which occurred in a group followed a one-to-one discussion with a silent member outside of the group. The facilitator took the tack of saying to the group members that they felt that they had more to offer in the group than was being seen and suggested that they volunteer themselves as the group chair. This validation of the member's worth in the group gave the student the confidence to push themselves into an unfamiliar role which they turned out to be very effective in and this was openly acknowledged by the other group members.

Understanding the effects of different personality types on the dynamics of PBL groups and learning how to manage them effectively is a skill which is required for both group members and facilitators as the impact they can have can be detrimental to the learning experience of the student. Baptiste (2003) discusses the role of self-assessment and reflection in PBL and it is important that students and facilitators become comfortable at reflecting on the impact of the self within PBL groups and are able to utilise this knowledge to manage themselves and others within the group environment. These transferable skills will prove to be invaluable in all work-based teams in the future.

Group commitment and motivation

A lack of commitment to the group is an issue often identified by students as causing difficulties within the PBL group (De Grave *et al.*, 2001; Hendry *et al.*, 2003). This can manifest itself in many different ways such as lateness, absenteeism, lack of preparation for tutorials, wanting to leave groups early and consistently offering to take the 'easy' option in terms of research. Levi (2007) adopts the term *social loafing* which can cause the biggest motivational problems in groups and teams. Social loafing occurs when there is a reduction of individual contributions when people work in groups and this can result in individuals' free loading off the group. This can be either because they do not think their contributions are valued or, more commonly, because they know that they will still benefit from the group's efforts regardless of their own input. It is natural within PBL groups that individuals' levels of contribution and commitment will vary over the life of the group but it becomes problematical when it is done consistently. Students report high levels of frustration with group members who do this but find it difficult to identify strategies for dealing with lack of commitment to the group (Hendry *et al.*, 2003). Not attending to this problem can lead the group to develop pairing and subgroups which will threaten the cohesiveness of the group and reinforce the lack of commitment as the more members value the membership of the group the more motivated they are to perform.

Levi (2007) suggests that to combat this phenomenon, groups need to enter into discussion about the effects of social loafing on the motivation of the group. He identifies that the most motivated and committed teams have clear goals, challenging tasks to complete, utilise group roles effectively and know how they are going to be evaluated and rewarded. Strategies which can be utilised to enhance group motivation and cohesiveness include the following:

▪ Use of a group learning contract which identifies both individual and group learning needs, resources to be used and evidences that learning needs have been met. Matheson (2003) reports that students felt that using a learning contract within PBL groups helped the group structure its thinking and provided an organisational system for the group.

▪ Group guidelines which explicitly lay out expectations of group members and can be used to reflect on group performance and motivation.

▪ Allocated group roles which should be rotated regularly.

▪ Regular evaluation and feedback on group performance which is particularly important if the PBL tutorial group work is not assessed summatively within the curriculum. It is human nature for students to be assessment driven, and formative self and peer assessment needs to be valued by both group members and facilitators for it to be effective (Brown *et al.*, 1994).

Dealing with conflict and group tension

Conflict within teams is a natural part of the group process (Levi, 2007) and is a theme which is often reflected upon by PBL group members, as one student reported:

it caused everyone to feel uncomfortable and just the silences were terrible, you know, we would all be sat there looking at the walls and it's not productive really . . . . . the tension was always there . . . .

It is rare to experience conflict in the first stage of group development as members are focused on understanding the PBL process and their role within the group. Communication tends to be polite, accommodating and avoidant of controversial issues; however, as groups develop into stage two disagreements about roles, goals and tasks begin to emerge and the culture of leadership and group structure will begin to be challenged. This stage of the group is seen as necessary and healthy as it helps groups to negotiate a unified direction following the emergence of divergent views.

Conflict can be a catalyst for groups to explore new approaches to problem solving; it can help members understand issues better and appreciate different views and perspectives and encourage creativity within groups (Wheelan, 2005; Levi, 2007). Feedback from students indicates that individuals learn more about themselves and others when there is tension within the groups than when groups are running smoothly. In fact, if conflict is absent in the life of a group, this can be an indicator that something is wrong such as a very dominant leader who suppresses any debate and dissent or a group that is working in a routine manner and not trying to improve its performance.

Groupthink is a type of group decision-making problem which can occur when the group's desire to maintain good relations becomes more important than reaching good decisions (Janis (1972) cited in Levi (2007)). When groupthink occurs, groups fail to look at alternative solutions, individuals do not express opinions if they differ from the group and there is suppression of negative comments in group discussions. This can limit problem solving and critical evaluation of decisions made by the group. Conflict, however, can be damaging to the group, particularly if it causes emotional distress to individuals and results in difficulties in communication.

Generally, teams do not handle conflict well because of misconceptions that conflict is bad and should be avoided (Levi, 2007) but if it can be accepted as a necessary group dynamic, this gives an opportunity to work constructively with it. Levi (2007) suggests that groups adopt an attitude of conflict management as opposed to conflict resolution as some conflicts will never be fully resolved. He suggests that a collaborative approach to conflict management is the most effective strategy which requires group members to be assertive and cooperative in negotiating acceptable strategies to problem solving.

In PBL groups it is rare for groups to require formal intervention in managing conflicts and many of the strategies previously discussed will be successful in dealing with difficulties that arise. Interestingly, feedback from students indicates that they believe issues should be dealt with within the group by the students themselves. They feel that this is most effective and recognise that this helps them develop useful skills in negotiation and learning to appreciate diversity within their groups. As a facilitator new to PBL, it can be tempting to feel that it is your role to facilitate conflict management but generally group members do tend to work issues out for themselves.

Transference in PBL groups

A final consideration relevant to PBL groups is the psychological process of transference and counter-transference, a therapeutic process normally recognised within psychotherapy groups. Transference is an unconscious process which occurs between group members where an individual responds to another individual in a manner based on past responses towards a significant person. Transference is most common towards the group leader who may or may not be the facilitator. Counter-transference occurs when the group leader responds in an uncharacteristic way towards a group member based on responses from his or her own past relationships. These complex dynamics are rarely acknowledged within PBL groups and PBL literature; there is a tendency to regard difficulties between group members and facilitators as *personality clashes*. It is useful for anyone working within PBL groups to have an awareness of these phenomena and Finlay (1993) and Yalom and Leszcz (2005) provide useful overviews.

Developing team working skills through PBL

Today's health and social care settings rely on and deliver their services through professional teams as do most modern organisations (Driskell *et al.*, 2006). As educators of health and social care professionals, educational providers have a duty to train graduates who are 'fit for practice' (Davys & Pope, 2006, p. 572). The ability to manage group dynamics within PBL groups is a vital skill for students to master in order to transfer effectively into multi-disciplinary and multi-agency teams upon graduation. Research by Reeves *et al.* (2004) suggests that PBL has positive benefits for occupational therapy (OT) graduates, particularly in the area of team-working abilities, as they move into their field of professional practice. Holen (2000), in relation to medical training, suggests that the PBL group gives the best chances for individuals to develop the social skills that will enhance professional relationships with both patients and fellow workers.

So what makes a good team player and how does this relate to skills developed in PBL groups? Driskell *et al.* (2006) outline a useful model of the 'Big Five' personality traits in relation to team effectiveness. In brief, these are emotional stability, extraversion, openness to experience, agreeableness and conscientiousness. These traits are further composed of more specific facets which are believed to be relevant to team effectiveness. Discussion with students links several of the underlying facets identified by Driskell *et al.* (2006) as being areas where they feel that they have developed through the PBL process.

Managing dominance behaviours in self and others is a common area which needs to be mastered, as effective team members need to be able to subjugate the desire for personal dominance within the group in order to work effectively as part of a mutually reliant team (Driskell *et al.*, 2006). One student describes the benefits of dealing with dominance within the group as a personal important learning point:

> I think I learned more from it [PBL] because it made me appreciate the
> fact that people are different and you are not always going to agree

but then there is a way of working through it.... Even at the times of uncomfortable feelings and tension you can get through it and come out with a productive outcome at the end. I think that was really good for me to appreciate because before doing this course I was always quite black and white and now I can look outside the box a bit and appreciate other people.

This also links to the facet of flexibility which is the ability and willingness to respond differently to different situations, a skill necessary to master within the PBL environment. Further areas of development recognised by students include the ability to develop trust in other people's work; learning how to delegate and recognising that others would produce work as good as their own; appreciation and tolerance of differences between group members and the development of diplomacy skills. All these areas are skills recognised within high functioning teams and are useful transferable skills which can be utilised in future work-based teams.

Robertson and Finlay (2007) and Lloyd *et al.* (2007) recognise both the challenges and support that can occur through team working, as faced by newly qualified OT graduates in their first posts. The PBL group appears to be a setting where students can develop skills necessary to function in today's challenging service settings.

Conclusion

This chapter focuses on the role of group dynamics within PBL groups and how the ability to manage group dynamics enables students to develop transferable team-working skills into professional practice. A model of group development was explored to illustrate how PBL groups may develop and common challenges in groups have been identified from a student and facilitator perspective. The most common difficulties facing those new to PBL are managing particular personality traits within groups, developing group commitment and motivation and managing group conflict and tension. Suggestions have been made as to how to manage these dynamics more effectively and the chapter concludes with a brief exploration of some of the benefits of PBL environments and student preparation for working in teams within health and social care practice.

References

Baptiste, S.E. (2003) *Problem-Based Learning: A Self–Directed Journey*. Slack Incorporated, NJ.

Brown, S., Rust, C. & Gibbs, G. (1994) *Strategies for Diversifying Assessment in Higher Education*. The Oxford Centre for Staff Development.

Corey, M.S. & Corey, G. (1997) *Group Processes and Practice*, 5th edn. Brooks/Cole Publishing Company, London.

Davys, D. & Pope, K. (2006) Problem based learning within occupational therapy education: a summary of the Salford experience. *British Journal of Occupational Therapy.* **69** (12), 572–574.

De Grave, W.S., Dolmans, D.H.J.M. & van der Vleuten, C.P.M. (2001) Student perceptions about the occurrence of critical incidents in tutorial groups. *Medical Teacher.* **23** (1), 49–54.

Driskell, J.E., Goodwin, G.F., Salas, E. & O'Shea, P.G. (2006) What makes a good team player? Personality and team effectiveness. *Group Dynamics: Theory Research and Practice.* **10** (4), 249–271.

Finlay, L. (1993) *Groupwork in Occupational Therapy.* StanleyThornes Ltd, Cheltenham.

Hayes, N. (1997) *Successful Team Management.* International Thomson Business Press, London.

Hendry, G.D., Ryan, G. & Harris, J. (2003) Group problems in problem-based learning. *Medical Teacher.* **25** (6), 609–616.

Holen, A. (2000) The PBL group: self-reflections and feedback for improved learning and growth. *Medical Teacher.* **22** (5), 485–488.

Janis, I.L. (1972) *Victims of Groupthink: A Psychological Study of Foreign–Policy Decisions and Fiascos.* Houghton Mifflin, Oxford.

Levi, D. (2007) *Group Dynamics for Teams*, 2nd edn. Sage Publications, London.

Lloyd, C., King, R. & Ryan, L. (2007) The challenge of working in mental health settings: perceptions of newly graduated occupational therapists. *British Journal of Occupational Therapy.* **70** (11), 460–470.

Matheson, R. (2003) Promoting the integration of theory and practice by the use of a learning contract. *International Journal of Therapy and Rehabilitation.* **10** (6), 264–269.

Reeves, S., Summerfield Mann, L., Caunce, M., Beecraft, S., Living, R. & Conway, M. (2004) Understanding the effects of problem-based learning on practice: findings from a survey of newly qualified occupational therapists. *British Journal of Occupational Therapy.* **67** (7), 323–327.

Robertson, C. & Finlay, L. (2007) Making a difference, teamwork and coping: the meaning of practice in acute physical settings. *British Journal of Occupational Therapy.* **70** (2), 73–80.

Tuckman, B.W. & Jenson, M.A.C. (1977) Stages in small group development revisited. *Group and Organizational Studies.* **2**, 419–427.

Wheelan, S.A. (2005) *Group Processes: A Developmental Perspective*, 2nd edn. Allyn and Bacon, London.

Yalom, I.D. & Leszcz, M. (2005) *The Theory and Practice of Group Psychotherapy*, 5th edn. Basic Books, New York, NY.

7: Assessing problem-based learning curricula

Sue Pengelly

Introduction

Other chapters have established the importance of developing quality learning and teaching to facilitate students to undertake self-directed learning and to develop as reflective practitioners for a broad range of health and social care professions. This chapter explores the powerful influence that assessment has on this learning experience and argues that it can either reinforce or undermine the principles of problem-based learning (PBL). It aims to highlight the essential nature of aligning the purpose and practice of assessment with both the aims and values of PBL and the learning needs of future professionals.

All through higher education (HE) increasing emphasis has been placed on the importance of establishing good quality teaching and learning environments but less on assessing students' learning (Knight, 2007). Learning and assessment have traditionally been seen as two distinct activities; this chapter emphasises the fundamental inter-relationship between the two.

> Assessment, rather than teaching, has a major influence on students' learning. It directs attention to what is important. It acts as an incentive for study. And it has a powerful effect on what students do and how they do it.
>
> (Boud & Falchikov, 2007, p. 3)

It is important to understand the purpose and practice of assessment as it has been contended that designing an assessment strategy which is fit for the purpose is the most useful thing a tutor can do to influence learning and teaching (Brown, 1999). This necessitates making considered decisions about the following questions.

- **Why are we assessing?**
  Is there clarity about the diverse range of reasons why students are assessed and an appropriate balance between the enhancement of learning and the accreditation for learning?

■ **What are we assessing?**
Is what is assessed consistent with how students learn on a PBL course and comparable with the requirements for professional practice?

■ **Who is best placed to assess?**
Are tutors maintaining unilateral control or are students accepted as adult self-directed learners and involved in assessment?

■ **How are we assessing?**
What methods are appropriate for use on professional PBL courses and what assessment practices are adopted related to marking, feedback and timing of assessment?

These issues will all be explored in greater detail throughout the chapter and positioned within the context HE, PBL and professional practice. The discussion will explore the power issues inherent in assessment and examine the challenges to implementing student-centred assessment while simultaneously ensuring fitness to practice.

Why are we assessing?

Before any consideration is given to what or how we might choose to assess, it is important to recognise the numerous and potentially conflicting reasons as to why we assess. Brown and Glasner (1999) acknowledged that assessment in HE matters to a broad range of interested parties for differing reasons. Their original list has been expanded to relate specifically to PBL degrees leading to a professional qualification within health and social care (Table 7.1).

In summary, assessment is undertaken to support, improve and measure learning and to assure standards (Savin-Baden & Howell Major, 2004).

A frequently used distinction categorises the main purposes of assessment as formative and summative assessment (Biggs, 1990).

■ **Formative** – to enhance learning with the focus of judgement being for the benefit of individual students. This is necessary to enable students to learn well.

■ **Summative** – for accreditation and to certify achievements with the focus of judgement being for the external world. This is essential to show eligibility to practice.

Another, less frequently used category which is of special relevance to both PBL and professional education is.

■ **Ipsative** – to measure how far individual students have moved in relation to their own previous learning and performance. This is required for continuous professional development (CPD).

There has recently been a move away from assessment *of* learning towards assessment *for* learning. Within PBL, importance is placed

Table 7.1 Reasons for assessment from diverse perspectives.

Students	■ to provide opportunities to construct and demonstrate their understanding of issues related to professional practice ■ to provide feedback on strengths and areas for development ■ to motivate their ongoing learning ■ to encourage self-reflection and engagement in continuing professional development (CPD) ■ to provide access to employment and career development
Tutors	■ to challenge students to develop as a professional ■ to provide feedback for student development ■ to identify students who need extra support ■ to evaluate and modify learning and teaching
Parents and significant others	■ to measure how students are progressing ■ to demonstrate fair and transparent procedures
Potential employees	■ to indicate who will make good all round employees
Clients	■ to certify that graduates can practise competently
Regulating and professional bodies	■ to demonstrate fitness to practice ■ to adhere to required ethical and practice standards
Educational institutions	■ to certify the achievement of individual students ■ to demonstrate robust systems ■ for quality assurance
Funders for HE	■ to demonstrate maintenance of standards
Subject reviewers, QAA	■ to demonstrate effective transparent systems

QAA, Quality Assurance Agency.
Adapted from Brown and Glasner (1999).

on formative assessment and designing summative assessments which maximise learning (Savin-Baden, 2003). However, this needs to be balanced with essential role of summative assessment, which 'converts learning into credentials' (Winter, 2003, p. 114). While formative and summative assessments were initially understood as separate categories, Brown (1999) suggested that it was more helpful to consider them as extreme ends of a continuum. In reality, every assessment combines elements of both and can be positioned at some point along that continuum.

With such a range of reasons for carrying out assessment it can clearly be a challenge to balance all of these potentially conflicting demands. A central discussion related to professional degrees revolves around the need to balance enhancement of learning with attaining a professional qualification. A useful extension to this debate is the concept of sustainable assessments, which are defined as

> assessment practices that met the needs of an institution to certify or provide feedback on students' work, but which would also meet the longer term need of equipping students for a lifetime of learning.
>
> (Boud & Falchikov, 2007, p. 7)

This challenges educators to adopt a longer term perspective on assessment, contending that the key purpose of assessments within university is to prepare individuals for a lifetime of learning and professional practice. This shift is clearly compatible with the importance placed upon ongoing personal and professional development within the context of health and social care professions, while the need for certification to demonstrate fitness for practice is also acknowledged.

Having identified the overt purposes of assessment, it is useful to recognise the existence of more covert reasons for assessment which can have a significant, potentially undermining effect on how students interpret and engage in assessment practices. Assessment is recognised to be a

> value laden activity surrounded by debates about academic standards, preparing students for employment, measuring quality and providing incentives.
>
> (Boud & Falchikov, 2007, p. 9)

As such assessment practices can serve to express institutional values through conveying hidden messages to students about what is actually important (Epstein & Hundert, 2002); this can reinforce or negate PBL and professional values. While one of the major purposes of assessment in HE is to enhance an appropriate level of learning, research suggested that assessment has a fundamental impact on whether students adopt deep or surface approaches to learning (Rust, 2002) and that it can be counterproductive by encouraging a narrow instrumental approach to learning (Biggs, 1990). Assessment practices also embody tutors' actual rather than espoused approaches to education, which range from being 'teacher focused and content orientated' to being 'student focused and learning orientated' (Entwistle, 2000, p. 5). Within PBL, tutors may espouse one approach to learning and teaching while revealing a more covert approach within the assessment practices they adopt.

Savin-Baden (2003, p. 102) reported that tutors rarely made it clear to students that 'assessment was part of their learning journey'. She also identified a range of dilemmas which may be present when assessing PBL courses. She warned against the danger of coded practices and unintended side effects of assessments which can undermine the intentions of even the most student centred tutors. She acknowledged that inherent power issues exist within assessments and argued that assumptions within assessments can undermine the PBL philosophy of responsibility and autonomy by determining what 'actually counts as knowledge and knowing in a given field' (Savin-Baden, 2003, p. 106).

Assessment systems can be resistant to change, especially when they 'unreflexively embody many socio-political assumptions about what education is for' (Boud & Falchikov, 2007, p. 9). As tutors on PBL courses leading to professional qualifications it is essential that we adopt a reflexive stance to assessment, to challenge assumptions behind our practice, develop overt decision-making and remain open to explore our students' perspective on the purpose and practice of assessment.

What are we assessing?

Having explored the diverse reasons for undertaking assessment, this section will consider what needs to be assessed to prepare students for their future professional practice while remaining consistent with PBL within the broader context of HE.

Within the professional context of health and social care education, assessment for certification has often been seen as paramount, with subsequent emphasis placed on assessing competencies including core knowledge and basic skills. This can focus attention on lower level achievements rather than the more complex ones required for professional practice (Knight, 2007). Taylor (1997) argued that the assessment of what is easily and reliably measured should be counterbalanced by valid assessment of abilities and skills, which are less easy to measure but remain essential to professional practice. A more holistic view of competencies is required, moving beyond behavioural outcomes which tended to divide theory from practice. Such a concept of competencies would relate required attributes (knowledge, attitudes, values and skills) to the professional context (Brew, 1995). Epstein and Hundert (2002, p. 226) defined professional competence as

> The habitual and judicious use of communication, knowledge, technical skills, clinical reasoning, emotions, values and reflection in daily practice for the benefit of the individual and community being served.

This approach should help to alleviate the danger of assessing competencies in isolation from the needs of individual learners or the contexts in which they are required. If competency statements are understood as 'relatively stable and static representations of a critically reflective dynamic creative process' (Brew, 1995, p. 61) they should be developed through ongoing dialogues with learners. This can prevent competency-based education from becoming competency-centred rather than student-centred. They must remain interlinked with both professional context and relevant knowledge base and a distinction drawn between transferable skills and the ability to transfer them (Savin-Baden & Howell Major, 2004). While word processing skills may be relatively straightforward to transfer between situations, group working skills are likely to be more context dependent.

In relation to PBL, Savin-Baden (2003) confirmed that the performative approach to awarding competencies was too narrow as it omitted the process of how students learn. In a study investigating students' perception of assessment on PBL courses, she reported that many students felt that much of their learning went unrewarded and there was a 'mismatch between the collaborative ethos of PBL and the outcome-focused assessment' (Savin-Baden, 2004, p. 230), which rewarded the individual rather than the group. Her research demonstrated the need to assess aspects which reflect PBL philosophy and how knowledge is constructed within specific professions in a way which remains contextualised and meaningful to students.

Research also revealed tensions between HE and the assessment of professional education. Emphasis is often placed on maintaining reliable academic standards in contrast to the development of personal and process knowledge which has higher consequential validity for future practice (Taylor, 1997). Any such inconsistencies can give students conflicting messages about what is important. The importance of ensuring that assessment is integral to course design and learning and teaching is increasingly recognised within HE. This has been supported by Bigg's influential concept of constructive alignment which emphasised the importance of consistency between expected learning outcomes, learning opportunities and assessments. Biggs (1999) explained that 'constructive' related to the learner's construction of meaning through learning activities and that 'alignment' related to the teacher's role in setting up appropriate learning activities and assessments to achieve and measure the intended learning outcomes. In this way he argued that

> All components of the system address the same agenda and support each other. The students are 'entrapped' in this web of consistency, optimising the likelihood that they will engage in the appropriate learning activities. I call this network *constructive alignment*.
>
> (Biggs, 1999, p. 64)

While tutors start with learning outcomes and culminate with assessment, learners often reverse that by initially focusing on assessment and ending with learning outcomes (Biggs, 1999). This is unproblematic if they are consistent, but inconsistencies result in students searching for the hidden curriculum revealed through assessment.

While constructive alignment has been critiqued as simply stating self-evident ideas (Winter, 2003) and as adopting an over simplistic approach to constructivism without exploring how a unity of understanding can be interactively achieved (Savin-Baden, 2003), it remains a useful concept to help identify and prevent potential inconsistencies. Biggs (1999, p. 71) stated that 'problem-based learning is alignment itself', especially within the context of professional teaching as objectives, learning and assessment all involve students solving profession-related problems (Biggs, 2003). However, he did qualify this by warning that cracks could appear if assessments which were inconsistent with the academic values of PBL were used (Biggs, 1990).

In the drive to ensure that assessments are consistent with both PBL and the needs of future professional practice it is suggested that emphasis is placed on

- the application and integration of a range of knowledge to professional problems;
- the process of learning and development of a personal understanding linked to future practice;
- reflective practice both as a learner and professional;
- clinical reasoning processes, problem solving and decision making within a range of professional settings;
- self-directed learning (meta-cognition, self-assessment and time management skills);
- ability to research and utilise a broad range of formal and informal resources;
- group working and communication skills (contribution to group learning, cooperation, negotiation, giving and receiving peer feedback);
- attitudes consistent with PBL and professional practice (value opinions of others and tolerate ambiguity);
- professional attitudes (responsible, ethical and person-centred);
- professional specific skills and
- emotional intelligence (acknowledge own emotions, responsiveness and caring for others).

Who should assess?

Tutors are encouraged to be mindful about power inherent in assessment and aware that unilateral assessment is inconsistent with the aim of autonomous learning. Within PBL, traditional views of authority and power have been overturned and this should include assessment. This often involves challenging attitudes and practices of learners and tutors who were socialised in educational systems dominated by unilateral assessment (Savin-Baden & Howell Major, 2004).

Within professional practice:

Assessments by peers, staff, expert practitioners and so on are essential in assisting learners to form sound judgements. Assumptions that learners are unable to make judgments undermine their capacity to do so.

(Biggs, 1990, p. 109)

The range of people available to undertake assessment can usefully include the following:

- Tutors – if subject expertise is needed
- Students – when reflection is required
- Peers – for effective formative feedback
- Practice educators – related to placement experience
- Clients – to encourage client-centred working

This section will focus specifically on self, peer and collaborative assessment as these offer opportunities to develop essential skills required by both PBL students and future professionals.

Self-assessment

Once learning is conceived as constructing rather than receiving information, self-assessment becomes a fundamental requirement for all learning through the process of reviewing the present position, identifying learning needs and evaluating whether these have been achieved (Boud, 1995). As such, Boud (1995) argued that self-assessment was central to effective learning within HE as it promoted student autonomy and meta-cognition, which are vital skills for ongoing learning. It is also an expected outcome linked to a future driven view of learning (Tan, 2007) and essential within professional education (Taylor, 1997).

> Because it is professionally imperative for nurses, for doctors, for teachers, for everybody, that you're able to realistically self assess . . . .That ability to self assess is the springboard for your life long learning.
>
> (Tan, 2007, p. 120)

Self-assessment is inter-related to reflection (Boud, 1995) through which professionals engage with the complex problems of the real world (Schön, 1987). Both self-assessment and reflective practice require the ability to think critically, plan and implement changes to practise and evaluate the effectiveness of those changes.

Self-assessment is embodied within all PBL courses either implicitly in the PBL process or more explicitly through specific assessments. This reflects the notion that self-assessment operates as both a verb (the ongoing process) and a noun (an individual event) (Boud, 1995). It reiterates the self-autonomy, responsibility, self-directed learning and critical monitoring skills encapsulated within PBL. While self-assessment can be empowering this is only the case when used appropriately, with the focus not simply on the introduction of self-assessment activity, but on the development of self-assessment ability (Tan, 2007). Self-assessment can initially be overwhelming for learners who lack the confidence to provide judgement (Taylor, 1997), so the development of emotional as well as cognitive abilities is necessary. Skills in self-assessment can be developed through the use of learning contracts, ongoing reflection and evaluating work against marking criteria.

Peer assessment

Peer assessment has clear links with working alongside other students in PBL and colleagues in professional practice. It is useful to distinguish between *inter-peer* assessment (by other members of the cohort) and *intra-peer* assessment (from within the group you have been working with). Both can provide timely feedback and the latter can help separate individual contribution from the group as a whole.

It involves having increased power and responsibility for supporting and judging other learners and, subsequently, has more potential hazards than self-assessment (Boud, 1995; Savin-Baden, 2003). Summative peer assessment can be unpopular and Boud (1995) argued that this is best avoided because it could decrease cooperation between students and cause feelings of resentment. In contrast, formative assessment is more acceptable to students as it has the potential to provide alternative perspectives and immediate feedback in a way which is less threatening than from a tutor. As few students have experience of peer assessment, they often need support, guidelines and opportunities to practise developing marking criteria and giving and receiving constructive feedback. Areas that are useful to peer assess include presentations to the cohort, contributions within tutorial groups and initial ideas for summative assessments. Academic posters can provide a useful initial focus for peer assessment and students can be facilitated to develop a range of criteria including, visual layout and impact; appropriateness for audience; and content and supporting evidence.

Collaborative assessment

Collaborative assessment recognises that no learning happens in isolation but occurs alongside peers, tutors and placement educators. This approach encourages mutual responsibility between several assessors. This can reduce the negative effects of unilateral assessment and progressively introduce greater student responsibility for assessment. A useful starting point can involve self and tutor assessment of a formative assignment, including a reflection on the work undertaken, and a tutorial to discuss each other's evaluation or to negotiate a grade using the same criteria (Savin-Baden, 2003). A combination peer and self-assessment can be combined in professional portfolio work and educator and self-assessment are often combined with feedback from other staff and clients in the placement setting. If used constructively, with the emphasis on iterative assessment rather than social comparison, this approach can increase motivation and self-esteem (Boud, 1995).

Self, peer and collaborative assessment are all effective approaches to use within professional PBL courses to enhance both present and future learning. Beyond that they can be transformative as they confront conventional ideas about the controlling role of assessment. Tan (2007) argued that self-assessment (which can be extended to include peer and collaborative assessment), is positioned within the emancipatory discourse of participation and interaction which encourages reflexivity in both learners and tutors. He identified three progressive concepts related to self-assessment moving from teacher driven (focused on pleasing the teacher); to programme driven (focused on completing the programme) and finally, future driven which focused on using the programme to prepare for future learning. Whereas the first two maintain existing assessment practices and emphasise reliability and consistency of marking between students and tutors (Boud, 1995), the third promotes a more critical and reflexive approach to learning and assessment and is the required level of engagement within both PBL and professional practice.

How are we assessing?

Having explored the diverse reasons for assessment, identified what needs to be assessed and explored the power issues inherent in considering who should assess, it is now useful to review some methods used to assess students on professional PBL degrees. Methods selected may well differ from those used on traditional courses which design assessments to assess the transfer of knowledge, based on the assumptions that knowledge is universal and that assessment can be objective and reliable. In contrast, PBL courses are based on the concept that knowledge is constructed and has multiple meanings which recognises the inter-relationship between the process and the product and acknowledges that assessment is subjective and value laden (Savin-Baden & Howell Major, 2004).

As one aim of assessment is to promote present and future learning, it is important to select methods which students see as being more than merely an academic exercise. Learners are most likely to see the relevance of assessments to themselves if the methods used are authentic, related to professional practice and offer individual choice (Rust, 2002). Rather than selecting traditional essay and examination tools, tutors and learners on PBL courses have the opportunity to explore creative alternatives relevant to PBL and future practice. They should offer increased student responsibility; focus of the process as well as the product of learning; promote collaborative learning and facilitate reflection and self-evaluation.

Literature related to assessment of PBL courses leading to a health and social care professional qualification identified a range of methods being used (Alavi & Cooke, 1995; Van Der Vieuten *et al.*, 1996; Challis, 1999; Nendaz & Tekian, 1999; Baume & Yorke, 2002; Cunnington, 2002; Epstein & Hundert, 2002; Savin-Baden, 2003; Klenowski *et al.*, 2006). These include the following:

▪ Individualised learning contracts in university and on placement
▪ Group assessments leading to creative presentations
▪ Progress testing
▪ OSCE (Objective Structured Clinical Evaluation)
▪ Learning journals and portfolios linked CPD
▪ Triple jump (a three-stage process focusing on identifying, undertaking and evaluating learning)
▪ Tripartite assessment (a group report and two individual submissions: their own research and an account of the team process linked to theory)
▪ Oral assessment to explore clinical reasoning
▪ Patchwork texts (varied pieces of writing around a theme which are united by a reflective commentary)

Because of the need to assess a broad range of integrated knowledge and professional competencies related to practice alongside the evaluation of the process of learning, no single assessment is sufficient (Nendaz & Tekian, 1999). Therefore, a combination of assessments should be selected to provide a comprehensive assessment strategy. Table 7.2 provides a brief comparison of the above methods of assessment in relation to the previously identified essential elements of assessment within a PBL course, which leads to a professional qualification. It should be recognised that, while several of the assessments may touch on more of these areas, the table highlights the dominant areas they focus upon.

While it is beyond the scope of this chapter to examine all of these, the triple jump, portfolio and patchwork texts will be explored further.

The triple jump was initially a popular assessment, developed in the mid 1970s to replicate the PBL tutorial process on a one- to- one-basis and involved students in

▪ discussing a new professional scenario and identifying leaning goals;
▪ investigating learning resources for a limited time period;
▪ discussing the case in the light of their new learning, and evaluating their own performance.

Evaluation of the triple jump valued it for focusing on the process of problem solving and self-directed learning but expressed concern that it related to a single case and required a high level of tutor input during the first and last stages of the process (Nendaz & Tekian, 1999; Cunnington, 2002; Savin-Baden, 2003).

Table 7.2 Comparison of methods of assessment.

Assessment	Relevance to PBL and professional practice				Advantages and disadvantages
	Focuses on the process of learning	Offers individual choice and responsibility	Professional skills – reflection, team working, etc.	Related to professional practice/authentic	
Learning contracts	✓	✓	✓	✓	Flexible but time consuming to negotiate – a weak contract impacts on the final work
Group presentations			✓	✓	Values team working but hard to assess individual contributions
Progress testing	✓				Tests progress in knowledge acquisition while minimising negative effects of assessment on learning
OSCE			✓	✓	Can test a broad range of professional skills but problem with logistics
CPD portfolios	✓	✓	✓	✓	Valued by students as a professional requirement. Can lack focus and be challenging to mark
Triple jump	✓				Developed specifically for PBL but only focuses on one area and time consuming for tutors
Tripartite assessment	✓		✓		Combines group and individual work and less time consuming than the triple jump
Oral assessment of clinical reasoning		✓		✓	Closely related to professional practice. Logistically challenging to run
Patchwork text	✓	✓	✓	✓	Very flexible offering choice and variety. Can be challenging to mark

The use of portfolios is currently widespread throughout professional courses, based upon the approach to ongoing professional development embodied within the post-qualification requirement for CPD. As such they are recognised and valued by students as being authentic assessments (Baume & Yorke, 2002). While they are often flexible in structure, they usually include a range of evidence from practice along with a reflective commentary. They have been recognised as providing a framework within which individual students can plan, evidence and evaluate their own learning in an autonomous, reflective manner, drawing upon their own experience and accommodating their individual learning styles (Challis, 1999). However, they also provide challenges. They are often very time-consuming to construct, there is a danger that quality is substituted for quantity and their individualised nature can make assessing them challenging for tutors (Challis, 1999). Their original purpose was to present a collection of work rather than provide a unified record of learning for assessment purposes and they often still lack unity or clarity of focus, so it is essential to ensure that expectations are both clarified and shared (Baume & Yorke, 2002; Klenowski *et al.*, 2006).

The patchwork text is a more recent assessment which is presented as having potential for further development and requiring evaluation within professional PBL courses. It has been defined as a sequence of short pieces of varied writing which are joined by a reflective commentary (Winter, 2003). Students gradually build up the patchwork text throughout the module and have opportunities to discuss their separate pieces with their peers. Winter (2003) argued that this reflects the process of learning, which occurs gradually over time, as students construct their own developing understanding. This method of assessment also fits well with PBL's emphasis on critique and self-questioning (Savin-Baden, 2003) as it encapsulates:

> a model of learning and teaching which is focused on dialogue, critical reflection, reflexivity, self-awareness and self-evaluation.
>
> (Winter, 2003, p. 119)

In addition, it focuses on the process of learning; student autonomy and choice; learning in dialogue with others to develop and validate learning and the importance of critical personal engagement and reflection. Patchwork texts also offer ongoing opportunities for formative peer assessment within a summative assessment and enable students to draw on their own experience and utilise a range of writing skills to encourage creative expression of their learning (Akister *et al.*, 2003; McKenzie, 2003). It has been argued that they overcome the lack of overall synthesis inherent in portfolios by combining the advantages of the essay (unified structure) with the individual reflection and focus on process of the portfolio (Savin-Baden, 2003; Winter, 2003). However, as an innovative assessment they can be anxiety provoking for students and challenging to mark (McKenzie, 2003).

Marking and timing

Having explored some examples of existing assessment methods, how assessment is carried out in terms of marking, feedback and timing will now be considered. The way assessments are graded has a powerful influence on students and marks can shift attention away from their own learning and development. There is also concern that norm referencing and allocation of marks, with associated rank ordering of students, leads to competitive rather than collaborative learning which is counterproductive to PBL (Alavi & Cooke, 1995; Savin-Baden & Howell Major, 2004). Biggs (2003) argued that this approach was based on fundamentally flawed thinking about assessment within education, originating from the use of the measurement model developed within psychology to study differences between individuals rather than using a criteria-referenced approach. This results in an overemphasis on issues around fairness and standardised conditions at the expense of enhancing individual learning. It also encourages students to pursue extra marks rather than critically engaging in the learning process. In contrast, criterion referenced marking with associated verbal feedback is more likely to encourage collaborative critical learning. Savin-Baden (2004) challenged people to alter their view of assessment; so, even failure can be regarded as part of the developmental process rather than a way of differentiating between those who can and those who cannot.

Marking innovative assessments, including portfolios and patchwork texts, will also be challenging to mark because assessment criteria for individualised and reflective work differ from traditional academic criteria (Akister *et al.*, 2003). They need to integrate experience with the aims of the module and to achieve a balance between personal and academic writing. While most tutors are familiar with marking and providing feedback on traditional assessments they will need to be open to reflect upon how these assumptions and practices may be inconsistent when marking more innovative assessments.

The final area for consideration of how we assess relates to the timing of assessments. Tutors familiar with PBL will be aware that there is often a period of adjustment for students starting to learn through PBL, and while formative assessment and feedback are essential during this time, the introduction of summative and innovative assessment too early could be threatening (McKenzie, 2003). This is especially important to consider in the context of widening participation to increase retention of non-traditional students. Students' workload also need to be taken into account to ensure this remains realistic and that timing of assessments are considered in relation to group work commitments to help minimise the risk of students experiencing these as conflicting demands (Rust, 2002; Savin-Baden, 2004). If assessments are to be used to enhance learning they need to be integrated throughout the course and linked to learning opportunities.

Conclusion

This chapter has acknowledged the powerful influence that assessment has on learning and recognised that it can either reinforce or undermine PBL and professional education. It has sought to highlight the importance of aligning the purpose and practice of assessment with both the aims and values of PBL and the learning needs of future professionals. It has explored reasons why we assess, the need for compatibility in what we assess, who is best placed to assess and methods of how we undertake assessment. This discussion has explored the diverse, potentially conflicting and sometimes covert purposes of assessment and examined the challenges to implementing student-centred assessment while simultaneously ensuring fitness to practice. Power issues inherent in assessment have been examined and it has been argued that unilateral assessment is counterproductive when aiming at autonomous ongoing learning. Self, peer and collaborative assessment have all been acknowledged as potentially empowering approaches to assessment and as fundamental requirements for PBL and lifelong learning. Encouragement was given to tutors to select methods of assessment which are authentic and relevant to professional practice; promote individual choice and increased student responsibility; focus of the process as well as the product of learning; promote collaborative learning and facilitate reflection and self-evaluation. Tutors and students on PBL courses leading to professional qualifications are encouraged to adopt a reflective stance to assessment; to challenge assumptions behind practice; to develop overt decision making and to remain open to examine or express the students' perspective to help ensure that the purpose and practice of assessment remains congruent with the aims and values of PBL and professional practice.

References

Akister, J., Illes, K., Maisch, M., *et al.* (2003) Learning from the Patchwork Text Process – a retrospective discussion. *Innovations in Education and Teaching International.* **40** (2), 216–226.

Alavi, C. & Cooke, M. (1995) Assessing problem-based learning. In: *Problem-based Learning in a Health Sciences Curriculum* (ed. C. Alavi), pp. 126–140. Routledge, London.

Baume, D. & Yorke, M. (2002) The reliability of assessment by portfolio on a course to develop and accredit teachers in higher education. *Studies in Higher Education.* **27** (1), 7–25.

Biggs, J. (1990) Assessment and the promotion of academic values. *Studies in Higher Education.* **15** (1), 101–111.

Biggs, J. (1999) What the student does: teaching for enhanced learning. *Higher Education Research and Development.* **18** (1), 57–75.

Biggs, J. (2003) *Aligning Teaching and Assessment to Curriculum Objectives.* Learning and Teaching Support Network Generic Centre, York.

Boud, D. (1995) *Enhancing Learning through Self Assessment*. Kogan Page, London.

Boud, D. & Falchikov, N. (2007) *Rethinking Assessment in Higher Education: Learning for the Longer Term*. Routledge, London.

Brew, A. (1995) What is the scope of self assessment? In: *Enhancing Learning through Self Assessment* (ed. D. Boud), pp. 48–62. Kogan Page, London.

Brown, S. (1999) Institutional strategies for assessment. In: *Assessment Matters in Higher Education: Choosing and Using Diverse Approaches* (eds S. Brown & A. Galsner), pp. 3–13. Kogan Page, London.

Brown, S. & Glasner, A. (1999) *Assessment Matters in Higher Education: Choosing and Using Diverse Approaches*. Kogan Page, London.

Challis, M. (1999) Portfolio-based learning and assessment in medical education. *Medical Teacher*. **21** (4), 370–386.

Cunnington, J. (2002) Evolution of student assessment in McMaster University's MD Programme. *Medical Teacher*. **24** (3), 254–260.

Entwistle, N. (2000) *Promoting deep learning through teaching and assessment: conceptual frameworks and educational contexts*. Paper Presented at Teaching and Learning Research Programme (TLRP) Conference, Leicester, Nov. 2000.

Epstein, R. & Hundert, E. (2002) Defining and assessing professional competence. *Journal of the American Medical Association*. **287** (2), 226–235.

Klenowski, V., Askew, S. & Carnell, E. (2006) Portfolios for learning, assessment and professional development in higher education. *Assessment and Evaluation in Higher Education*. **31** (3), 267–286.

Knight, P. (2007) Grading, classifying and future learning. In: *Rethinking Assessment in Higher Education* (eds D. Boud & N. Falchikov), pp. 72–86. Routledge, London.

McKenzie, J. (2003) The student as an active agent in a disciplinary structure: introducing the patchwork text in teaching sociology. *Innovations in Education & Teaching International*. **40** (2), 152–160.

Nendaz, M. & Tekian, A. (1999) Assessment in problem-based learning medical schools: a literature review. *Teaching & Learning in Medicine*. **11** (4), 232–243.

Rust, C. (2002) The impact of assessment on student learning: how can research literature practically help to inform the development of departmental assessment strategies and learner-centred assessment practices? *Active Learning in Higher Education*. **3** (2), 145–158.

Savin-Baden, M. (2003) *Facilitating Problem-based Learning: Illuminating Perspectives*. Society for Research into Higher Education and Open University, Maidenhead.

Savin-Baden, M. (2004) Understanding the impact of assessment on students in problem-based learning. *Innovations in Education and Teaching International*. **11** (2), 223–233.

Savin-Baden, M. & Howell Major, C. (2004) *Foundations of Problem-based Learning*. Society for Research into Higher Education and Open University, Maidenhead.

Schön, D. (1987) *Educating the Reflective Practitioner*. Jossey-Bass, San Francisco.

Tan, K. (2007) Conceptions of Self-Assessment: What is Needed for Long-term Learning? In: *Rethinking Assessment in Higher Education* (eds D. Boud & N. Falchikov), pp. 114–127. Routledge, London.

Taylor, I. (1997) *Developing Learning in Professional Education*. The Society for Research into Higher Education and Open University Press, Buckingham.

Van Der Vieuten, C., Verwijnen, G. & Wijnen, W. (1996) Fifteen years of experience with progress testing in problem-based learning curriculum. *Medical Teacher*. **18** (2), 103–109.

Winter, R. (2003) Contextualising the patchwork text: addressing problems of coursework assessment in higher education. *Innovations in Education and Teaching International*. **40** (2), 112–122.

Part 2

The Theoretical Interface with Problem-Based Learning

8: Reflection and the problem-based learning curriculum

Gail Boniface

Introduction

This chapter offers a definition of reflection, outlining the essence of reflection as enabling the covert to be made overt. It argues that the purpose of reflection is to encourage professionals to go beyond mere evaluation of their practice. The chapter also links the process of problem-based learning (PBL) to reflection and vice versa, with the intention of discussing how the important aspect of clinical reasoning in a profession can be encouraged via reflection and the ways in which 'how to reflect' is learnt. Both of these issues are central to PBL. The chapter itself is based on research into reflection with practitioners and with first-year students following a PBL curriculum.

Defining reflection

Despite the development of numerous models of reflection (Mezirow, 1981; Boyd & Fales, 1983; Boud *et al.*, 1985; Gibbs, 1988; Johns, 2002; De Cossart & Fish, 2005), the nature of reflection remains nebulous and difficult to define. Thus it is also difficult, both to learn and to teach, yet it is an essential part of both developing practice and PBL. In order to consider how it may be learnt, taught or its prerequisite skills acquired, it is necessary to attempt to define it.

Reflection can be viewed as a structure for thinking (Dewey, 1933; Polyani, 1967), an emancipatory, evolutionary process (Habermas, 1974) and a structure for action (Mezirow, 1981; Fish *et al.*, 1991). Schön (1983, 1987) has been closely associated with the term, coining the phrases 'reflection in...' and 'reflection on action'. The overriding issue associated with reflection is that it is a good thing in itself (Boyd & Fales, 1983), whilst difficult to define and use (Boud *et al.*, 1985).

As far as structuring reflection is concerned, the content of reflection initially focuses on action by describing it. Including the description, the stages of reflection vary from Schön's two (Greenwood, 1998), Boud *et al.*'s three (1985), through Kolb's four (1984) to Boyd and Fales' six (1983). In general, despite the apparent discrepancy in the numbers of the stages of reflection, the writers agree on a number of main issues. Firstly, for the reflection to occur, the individual has to be open to reflection (Moon, 1999). Secondly, the feelings aroused by the event reflected upon should be recognised and dealt with (Kelly, 1994). Finally, the learning which occurs as a result of the reflection should be identified and turned into action (Kemmis, 1985). Reflection is also seen as consisting of different levels (Habermas, 1974; Van Manen 1977; Mezirow, 1981). The lowest level is the description of the event being reflected upon. The highest levels lead to the reflective person recognising and challenging the 'assumptions underlying' (Brookfield, 1993, p. 13) his or her beliefs and action. This aspect of reflection is rather nebulous, but seen as essential.

Colaizzi (1973) views the need for the person reflecting to understand his or her own reflective ability. Horowitz (1978, p. 36) encapsulates both the circular nature of reflection and its self-revelatory nature with the following comment:

> Reflective self awareness is the sense of being the thinker of one's thoughts.

Thus, as McGill and Beatty (1993, p. 8) comment 'reflectivity can be profound or superficial'. This aspect of reflection's nature brings up the issue of evaluation of practice at the lower reflection level or evaluation of self, within practice, at the deeper reflection level. Considering the espoused benefits of reflection, it is not surprising that the modern day professional is encouraged to become reflective and demonstrate reflective practice. Such skill in reflection is viewed as necessary in order for the professional to be regarded as able to respond flexibly to his or her changing working environment. If, however, this view of reflection is only related to the workplace action, not the professional taking the action, it can result in reflection being limited to evaluation of practice. Taylor (2000, p. 120) takes this kind of view of reflection as evaluation by seeing it as:

> describing an event and then looking at the decision-making process which underpins the actions taken within that event.

Reflection should include evaluation of practice or student learning, but it should also be more than that and lead to an entirely new definition of the practitioner or learner, via self-reflection: a self-reflection that leads to dealing with affective issues and confirming or challenging one's belief system (Barnett, 1997). Such a challenging of one's belief system should enable the practitioner to decide what type of practitioner he or she is and how content he or she is with that conclusion. Obviously, this type of self-reflection can be very liberating, but can also lead to discontent and considerable change in the way the practitioner works or the student learns. It can even lead to a change of job or career, if the reflector views the workplace as implacable and unchangeable. Advocating the need for reflection among professionals, Schön (1983) felt that professionals should not simply be solving problems with tried and tested professional responses. He also felt that they should actually be deciding what the nature of those problems are, via their use of technical skills, but also personal values and beliefs, which are open to change and challenge. The reflective practitioner and PBL learner is seen as one who is able to understand and, better still, to articulate his or her intuitive practice in relation to those problems he or she 'frames' (Schön, 1983, p. 210) and relate this to his or her view of himself or herself as a practitioner or learner. Thus becoming a reflective practitioner means we have to see ourselves as more than a person, asking ourselves 'how did I do that, was it right, was it wrong, how could I do it differently?'. We should turn ourselves into a practitioner who asks all those questions but adds, 'what ought I do now?'. As such a reflective practitioner, the ought is influenced by our personal judgement, our affective responses to the situation, our view of ourselves as a professional and our personal experience.

This introduction is intended to identify the main facets of reflection. It is also intended to suggest the reasons why reflection might be an important issue to us as thinking professionals rather than simply because it is required of us in our practice or in our learning. The connection between reflection and the ways in which professionals learn to reflect and use reflection in practice will be expanded upon below. Firstly, it is important to consider the models of reflection commonly used by heath and social care professionals.

Models of reflection

Boyd and Fales (1983) define reflection as a process with an outcome of a changed conceptual perspective on the part of the person reflecting. This is much deeper than seeing reflection as evaluation of our actions. Their model is concerned with explaining the process of reflection and linking it with learning. It contains a quotation which we can probably all recognise in ourselves: 'I know that I reflect and I consider myself a reflective person, but I have never thought about it and I am not exactly sure what it is that I do' (p. 103). They describe the process of reflection as one where it is necessary to define reflection for oneself and to be fully aware of when one is reflecting and actively trying to control the process.

They describe stages of reflection as

▪ a sense of inner discomfort;
▪ identification of clarification of the concern;

- openness to new information from internal and external sources, with ability to observe and take in from a variety of perspectives;
- resolution expressed as 'integration', 'coming together', 'acceptance of self reality' and 'creative synthesis';
- establishing continuing of self with past, present and future;
- deciding whether to act on the outcome of the reflective process undergone.

Thus, there seems to be a change occurring in the individual who reflects, but not necessarily in their action. Reflection, therefore, is more than evaluation of one's actions; it is an acceptance of oneself in relation to one's actions and a decision-making process as to whether one is content with that acceptance or not.

Often we reflect on negative events (perhaps encouraged by consideration of what we call critical incidents). Boyd and Fales' (1983) view of reflection should enable us to also reflect on positive events and really decide what made them positive and how we can build on that positivity. Presumably, if when we reflect we are not content with our actions and decision-making we change them both, but if we are content with them, we retain the values and consequential actions stemming from those values. What reflection offers us is a way of making those processes open and known to us. Reflection in Boyd and Fales' (1983) view, therefore, is not a stick with which to beat ourselves, but an articulation of our understanding of ourselves, and a process by which we can come to conclusions about ourselves, which may or may not necessitate change. Indeed it seems as if simply going through the process of reflection itself increases our reflective ability, 'the mere naming of the process – the bringing to consciousness of what is done naturally – is a significant aid to the use of reflective learning' (p. 113).

Fish and Twinn (1997) along with Purr, developed the strands of reflection model over a period of years from 1991 on. Their model is very popular with occupational therapists, but Fish has since developed it much further with Coles (Fish & Coles, 1998) and De Cossart (De Cossart & Fish, 2005). The original version talked about the following:

> Strands of reflection rather than levels allowed us to think about reflection in less of a hierarchical way than the word level implies. It was also appropriate to use the word strands to imply a rope, where the individual strands wrapped around each other to form something strong. This gave the impression that the strands were to be used in an interconnected way. Although, as you will see from the content of the strands, the first one, where the incident is described, needed to come first or there would have been nothing to reflect about.

These strands were the following:

1. **Factual strand** – set the scene and decide what was important in the event we are describing.

2. **Retrospective strand** – consider the whole thing and see what patterns and meanings we can find in it.
3. **Sub stratum strand** – seriously consider our assumptions and beliefs around what we think happened and why – this is the strand within which prejudices can be tackled.
4. **Connective strand** – the last strand asks us to consider what has been learnt from the event as a whole. How has it related to our past experience and what effect will it, should it, have on our future ones.

Although the strands are often still used, it is also worth considering Fish's new ideas on in-depth thinking and reflection with Coles (2005). Here, they represented reflective practice via the concept of an iceberg where the true expert practitioner is one who:

> knows something of what lies beneath the surface of his or her practice, and spends time and effort not just understanding it but developing it further, and who can then talk about it more publicly too.
>
> Fish and Coles (2005, p. 306)

The iceberg elements which are under the water (feelings, expectations, assumptions, attitudes, beliefs and values), can be in danger of being overwhelmed by the observable elements of the iceberg. Thus, this visible part of professional practice or what Fish and Coles (2005, p. 305) describe as 'our busyness' can overload the iceberg so that it topples over. Thus, they emphasise the importance of making the unseen elements of professional practice more overt and emphasise the importance of reflecting on them.

In De Cossart and Fish (2005), the iceberg analogy is continued and although the strands of reflection are present, a more complex definition of reflection and professional thinking is offered. Within this, the thread of personal professional judgement runs through clinical reasoning and decision-making, and it is this personal professional judgement which needs to be deconstructed and understood via reflection.

In both Fish and Coles (2005) and De Cossart and Fish (2005), the environment in which the reflection occurs is seen as of paramount importance, much as Schön (1987) discusses the reflective practicum, as an ideal location for reflection. Gibbs (1988) seems to have developed a model popular with nurses in particular. It originated (as did a number of these models) in education and is based on Kolb's Experiential Learning Cycle. It is very simple and consists of the following six phases:

1. Description of the event.
2. Feelings associated with it.
3. Evaluation – what was good and bad about the experience?
4. Analysis – what do the good and bad bits mean to you – what sense can you make of them?

5. Conclusion – problem solving question – what else could you have done?
6. Action plan – what would you do if it happened again?

Described simplistically, there seems little room in this model for a change of attitude or overall belief system, although, for the in-depth reflector, such self-reflection is always possible within any model.

Mezirow's (1981) model has layers of reflectivity which he calls levels. This may well imply a hierarchy. In the centre are the objects of reflectivity – take this to mean the things upon which we reflect. Then there are two outer layers: (i) consciousness and (ii) critical consciousness. It seems that the difference between them is that (i) is a level of awareness about the things upon which we are reflecting, whereas (ii) is at a level of reflecting on our reflecting. It would seem that it is at the (ii) level that we are open to transform or confirm our whole belief system, if that is what our reflection leads us to. The previous layers in the consciousness (ii) area would seem to encourage us to question how we have now arrived at our critical evaluation of those actions, thinking and beliefs. Each of the two main areas – consciousness and critical consciousness are split into separate levels.

Johns' (1994) model offers actual questions we may wish to ask ourselves whilst involved in reflection, although it also tends to imply that reflection is part of a larger evaluation process. The 'cues' Johns suggests we use seem to be stages of reflection in much the same way that Fish and Twinn's (1997) strands of reflection were. The model follows a similar format as follows:

1. Description.
2. Reflection (in this sense, a looking back over what it was that one was trying to do and asking, what were the consequences of that action?).
3. Influencing factors – you could read environment in here.
4. Alternative strategies – here comes the problem solving bit.
5. Learning – what have I learnt from this and what can I do in future instances?

Later, Johns (2000) developed his model into the model of structured reflection (MSR). In this, he wants the reflector to answer up to 16 specific questions. He has continued (2002, p. 10) to test 'the adequacy of the MSR to guide practitioners' and feels (2002, p. 13) that it is important to make 'connections between feelings and events', much as Fish and Twinn did earlier (1997). Unfortunately, Johns' (2002, p. 17) model has been seen as prescriptive (probably due to the specific questions) despite Johns' assertion that the model 'is not a prescription for reflection'. Indeed, Johns' comment concerning the prescriptive way in which models can be used, should remind us to use models flexibly.

Reflection, clinical reasoning and continuing professional development

A number of writers link reflection with clinical reasoning (Cohn, 1989; Mattingly, 1991; Schell & Cervero, 1993; Strong *et al.*, 1995; Crabtree & Lyons, 1997; Mason, 1999; Unsworth, 2004). Here, clinical reasoning is seen as more than having a reason for one's decisions (Mattingly, 1991). Clinical reasoning can be seen as consisting of three distinct aspects (Schell & Cervero, 1993): scientific reasoning where reasoning is located in the high hard ground of technical rationality; narrative reasoning, where reasoning is located in Schön's (1983) swampy lowlands; and pragmatic reasoning which owes much to reasoning strongly influenced by the workplace environment in which it takes place. Obvious links can then be made between clinical reasoning and reflection. Pragmatic reasoning becomes evaluation of practice and scientific reasoning utilises the practice skills, rather than the personal professional attributes required in narrative reasoning and reflection. Thus, when students within a PBL curriculum on a professionally based course are learning to clinically reason, they should also be learning to reflect and utilise their reflections within clinical reasoning.

Coppard *et al.* (1997, p. 35) see the use of the reflective process with students as a means of encouraging continued professional development and learning, later in professional life:

> The reflective process maintains a practitioner's active pursuit of knowledge

They also describe the need for a supportive environment if reflection is to be encouraged in students (see below).

Reflection in an educational context

Literature on adult learning often refers to the importance of reflection (Mezirow, 1981). Ideas about andragogy (Knowles *et al.*, 2005) in contrast to pedagogy imply the need for the (usually adult) learner to take responsibility for his or her learning and particularly to learn from experience. Such andragogical ideas are central to PBL and its positive sister, appreciative inquiry (AI) (Chapter 12). Kolb's (1984) learning cycle actually includes the word reflection. Boud and Walker (1990) view reflection as a 'vital element in any form of learning' (p. 8).

Views of learning as stemming from the individual learner's 'style' of learning describe a deep and surface style or approach to learning. Entwistle and Ramsden (1983) link these styles to the personality of the learner. It is plausible to identify similarities between a deep approach or style of learning and reflection; while a surface style or approach to learning, leans much more towards a mechanistic, technical way of approaching learning. There would also seem to be a connection between the nature of the learning and the environment in which it occurs. For example, the nature of the curriculum in which reflection is expected to occur would need to create an environment within which reflection is encouraged and valued, as PBL curricula claim they do. Gould and Taylor (1996) see not only the learner, but also the profession being learnt (in their instance, Social Work) as being at a disadvantage in many educational establishments. This disadvantage occurs because the nature of the practice being learnt is 'fuzzy' (p. 4). The 'fuzziness' of the profession to be learnt can be viewed as reminiscent of Schön's (1983) 'swampy lowland' (p. 42). Here, Schön describes the situations the professional has to deal with as 'confusing "messes" incapable of technical solution' (p. 42) and the professional as using experience, intuition, artistry as well as learnt techniques in order to act. Reflection, by its very nature, utilises and encourages all of these attributes or skills and is, therefore, very appropriate for learners on professional courses to learn. The issue to be addressed is how that learning is expected to occur. Reflection surely cannot be learnt in a rote way and needs to be relevant, experienced and encountered at the student's own pace. Again, these are all aspects which PBL curricula would claim to encompass.

Atkins and Murphy (1993) and Paterson (1995) view reflection as something that requires certain skills, both cognitive and affective. They suggest these skills are 'self awareness, description, clinical analysis, synthesis and evaluation' (p. 1190). The issue to address is, are these skills innate or can they be taught, or at least encouraged, in order to develop reflective ability? Reflection is also seen as a major component of learning (Kolb, 1984) and something that can be carried out alone or with others (Saylor, 1990), as well as a major component of professional development. It is also something which is central to PBL. Therefore, using reflection as well as teaching it on PBL curricula which educate developing professionals, should logically lead to that professional development.

Perhaps due to the vagueness of its definitions, reflection can appear complex and new (despite Dewey's discussion of it in 1933) to those being asked to reflect. Boyd and Fales' (1983) research responses suggested it is 'a spontaneous mental process that went on *(for their subjects)* without being controlled' (p. 104). Either of these views of reflection would make it very difficult to teach, yet it is seen as an important element in professional education and, particularly, in PBL.

There is a great connection between reflection and professions. Boyd and Fales' participants could all be described as experienced professionals, yet they were ambivalent towards the concept of reflection, sometimes seeing it as 'unwanted' (Boyd & Fales, 1983, p. 104) or uninvited. They even regarded it as intrusive and something which was uncomfortable and needed to be turned off. The respondents' replies suggested that the conscious recognition of the existence of the subject of reflection, similar to Freire's 'conscientizacao' or conscientization

(Freire, 1973), actually brought it about. Therefore, the first step to becoming reflective is to recognise reflection in the way Nystrand (1977) suggests one should 'name' or identify a process and value it in order to understand it. One can then learn how to use it. As Boyd and Fales (1983) state 'the mere naming process – the bringing to consciousness of what is done naturally is a significant aid to the use of reflective learning' (p. 113). Schön (1983) continues this theme by talking about 'naming and framing' (p. 42) in relation to problem identification, within the context in which problems occur. Rather than simply dealing with a problem, the professional has to first of all decide what the problem is, what form it takes and in what context it should be viewed. The connection between reflection and making the most of experience is strongly made by Kolb (1984) and Boud and Walker (1990). Kolb's Learning Cycle, used by Gibbs (1988), contains a reflective element. He also felt that Argyris and Schön's (1974) view was that,

> learning from experience is essential for individual and organizational effectiveness and that learning can occur only in situations where personal values and organizational norms support action based on valid information, free and informed choice, and internal commitment.
>
> (Kolb, 1984, p. 11)

The implication here is that learning from experience via reflection can be encouraged or inhibited by the atmosphere within which it is carried out – an atmosphere which is also crucial to a positive experience of PBL.

Teaching and assessing reflection in a problem-based learning curriculum

In his book, *Educating the Reflective Practitioner*, Schön (1987) describes the 'reflective practicum' (p. 157). Schön's (1987) view of such a practicum is an environment, which mirrors the 'messy situations' (p. 157) the professional needs to be able to perform in. At the same time, the practicum provides the stimulus for that professional to learn from that performance, in a reflective manner. Within such a reflective practicum, Schön (1987) believes the process of acquiring the 'design like artistry of professional practice' (p. 158) is 'learnable, coachable, but not teachable' (p. 158). The implication here is that learning from experience via reflection can be encouraged or inhibited by the atmosphere within which it is carried out. PBL curricula frequently use triggers, which mirror the 'messy situations' (Schön, 1987, p. 157) of the practice environment and probably offer a close facsimile of Schön's reflective practicum, which he views as central to learning to reflect. Kolb (1984) feels that it is important to take the environment into account in relation to learning and, therefore, in relation to reflection. Boud and

Walker (1990) continue the link between reflection and learning from experience, viewing:

> the idea of reflection as one of the key processes in learning from experience
>
> (p. 61)

During an action research project carried out with first-year undergraduate students of occupational therapy at two separate universities in 2005, the issues of teaching, learning and assessing reflection were addressed. Within that study, the students were concerned with the environment within which the reflection was expected to occur and related this to the environment within which PBL flourished. Students in both universities said that they reflected better when they felt the need to reflect and baulked against false situations where they felt reflection was forced upon them. Thus, when the reflection was externally imposed, it descended to the lower level of evaluation rather than reflection. They also linked assessing reflection to the truthfulness or falseness of the reflection, feeling that formally assessing the reflection created a danger of superficial or even false or made-up reflections. Reflective diaries, when assessed (Richardson & Maltby, 1995), have been shown to create exactly such an effect.

However, students do have a tendency (even those on PBL courses) to concentrate less on aspects of the curriculum which are not formally assessed, and it should be recognised that if reflection is a crucial part of PBL, which I believe it to be, then a way of assessing it as a process or product should be sought. My inclination is to assess the process formatively and encourage students to peer assess the product by considering the ways in which they have structured their portfolios, with a final summative assessment of students' reflections on their reflective content, rather than assessing the actual reflections. I have arrived at this conclusion because if I knew my reflections themselves were to be assessed, I know I would fabricate them into a format which I felt the assessors would like! Whereas, if I could *use* those reflections to create a more academic discussion of my learning about and use of reflection, I would be much more likely to be truthful. Thus, perhaps, reflection as a crucial element in PBL curricula, needs to be assessed in a more staged way:

- Self-assessment of the actual reflection
- Peer assessment of the way the reflection is structured
- Formal (summative) assessment of the student's discussion of their learning about reflection, where the raw reflective content (which is often too personal and even emotive to be assessed anyway) is the catalyst for reflection on reflective learning rather than the focus of assessment

If such stages were followed, it would be less likely that the comments, such as 'that was a good reflection' would be suffered, as experienced by students at the two universities researched. After all, how can an assessor external to the student or the situation possibly comment on the goodness or otherwise of the student's very personal view? Whereas, it would seem quite legitimate to comment on the academic way in which that personal reflection had been used in learning, such a staged and clear way of assessing reflection in a PBL curriculum would also help to deal with the considerable anxieties and vulnerability which students feel when *forced* to have their reflections assessed. It would also demonstrate that the environment in which the students were learning to reflect was a reflective one itself which trusted its students. This way of assessing reflection in the PBL setting may mean it could not be assessed until later on in the curriculum, as students would need to develop the reflective skills before being assessed on their use. Finally, reflection can be seen in the following three ways, all of which a PBL curriculum would wish to encourage:

1. Reflection as analysis of your professional performance to justify professional decision-making
2. Reflection as a way of confirming or testing your learning
3. Reflection as your process of personal development through internally exploring yourself as a learner or professional

Thus, reflection should be an integral learning tool within a PBL curriculum with the intention of encouraging its continuation in the professional life after qualification.

Time for reflection

An issue in reflection is the *time* needed to engage with the process, but also the timing of that reflection. Reflection comes about because of a need to reflect, not because we are told when we should reflect. PBL curricula allocate time to students to investigate triggers and must also offer time to students to reflect on those triggers, their reactions to them and their individualised learning, whilst at the same time recognising that different students will need to reflect at different times. To force reflection at times which suit the curriculum or in many professional courses, the practice placement, runs the risk of creating students who reflect by numbers or superficially. Yet, by not allocating time to reflection, the PBL curriculum would be negating its duties to encourage reflection. Thus, balancing the tensions created by different students' needs for time and timing is not easy. However, it is crucial if PBL is to encourage and *use* reflection, rather than assume it is happening. Much as models of reflection should be used flexibly, PBL curricula should timetable and use reflection flexibly as well.

The reflective environment

Coppard *et al.* (1997) described the environment within which reflection occurred (and by extrapolation learnt) as something which should be given serious consideration. Such a supportive environment is described as one which provides time, safety, good rapport, collaboration and structure, to enable reflection to occur (as opposed to forcing it into a timetable). These are all prerequisites for successful delivery of and engagement in a PBL curriculum. Carnall (1998) describes an attempt by an occupational therapy course to set up a reflective practicum (or environment) and the use of both a reflective portfolio and self and peer appraisal to encourage reflective ability in students. Within such an environment, the use of another person with whom to reflect is recommended, as long as the person reflecting feels supported while reflecting. Accepting, therefore, that reflection should probably be shared, the important issue of how to create the opportunity not only for the reflection, but also for the sharing to take place within a supportive environment, must be considered. Personally, reflecting with others who do not display evidence of valuing that reflection would be an unpleasant experience, unlikely to be repeated. As to me, reflecting on one's actions, let alone one's feelings and beliefs, creates a position of vulnerability, which requires a great deal of trust to overcome. Thus, the culture of the environment in which the reflection and reflective learning is to take place is important. If reflection is insisted upon, yet the opportunities and time to engage in it are not made available, the reflection will at best be superficial. Once all of these aspects related to an appropriate reflective environment are considered, it can be seen that they also should apply to and be found within a PBL curriculum. Thus, encouraging reflection in a PBL curriculum should be a natural occurrence if not an easy one.

Conclusion

There are, as can be seen, a number of models of reflection we can use as structures for our active reflection. There are a number of messages from all of them, which can be summed up as in order to use reflection in a useful manner, we need to overtly identify both our reflection and the manner in which we reflect. Once we have done that, we can then internalise the model(s) so that it becomes part of our way of thinking and consequently retain an organisation and useful structure to our reflection. We can also learn how to use models flexibly and not become constrained by them. It is otherwise too easy to say 'oh yes of course

I reflect' when all we actually do, is evaluate our work. We need to remind ourselves that true reflection goes further than this. It should, for example, require us to consider our belief system and whether we do or do not need to change it. We must also remember to reflect on good as well as bad experiences, as it is too easy to beat ourselves with reflections on bad events whilst ignoring or taking for granted, good ones.

The place of reflection in a PBL curriculum is central, as we would encourage our students to address all of the above issues. Both reflection and PBL, along with its positive sister AI, require the student to consider himself or herself as central to the learning, as a tool in the learning and as a thinking adult learner fully capable of reflecting on the learning which he or she participates in. However, the provider of the PBL curriculum needs to be very clear that both PBL and reflection will only flourish in an environment where reflection is valued and overt, rather than coercively insisted upon.

References

Argyris, C. & Schön, D.A. (1974) *Theory in Practice*. Jossey Bass, San Francisco, CA.

Atkins, S. & Murphy, K. (1993) Reflection: a review of the literature. *Journal of Advanced Nursing*. **18** (6), 1188–1192.

Barnett, R. (1997) *Higher Education: A Critical Business*. Society for Research into Higher Education and Oxford University Press, Oxford.

Boud, D., Keogh, R. & Walker, D. (1985) *Reflection: Turning Experience into Learning*. Kogan Page, London.

Boud, D. & Walker, D. (1990) Making the most of experience. *Studies in Continuing Education*. **12** (2), 61–80.

Boyd, E.M. & Fales, A.W. (1983) Reflective learning: key to learning from experience. *Journal of Humanistic Psychology*. **23** (2), 99–117.

Brookfield, S.D. (1993) *Developing Critical Thinkers. Challenging Adults to Explore Alternative Ways of Thinking and Acting*. Open University Press, Milton Keynes.

Carnall, L. (1998) Developing student autonomy in education: the independent option. *British Journal of Occupational Therapy*. **61** (12), 551–555.

Cohn, E. (1989) Fieldwork education. Shaping a foundation for clinical reasoning. *American Journal of Occupational Therapy*. **43** (4), 240–244.

Colaizzi, F. (1973) *Reflection and Research in Psychology: A Phenomenological Study of Learning*. Kendall Hunt, Dubee que, IA.

Coppard, B.M., Jensen, G.M. & Custard, C.L. (1997) Teaching reflection. Integrating clinical reasoning with narrative cases. *Occupational Therapy Practice*. **2** (12), 30–35.

Crabtree, M. & Lyons, M. (1997) Focal points and relationships: a study of clinical reasoning. *British Journal of Occupational Therapy*. **60** (2), 57–64.

De Cossart, L. & Fish, D. (2005) *Cultivating a Thinking Surgeon*. tfm Publishing, Shrewsbury.

Dewey, J. (1933) *How We Think*. D.C. Heath and Company, Boston, MA.

Entwistle, N. & Ramsden, P. (1983) *Understanding Student Learning*. Croom Helm, London.

Fish, D. & Coles, C. (1998) *Developing Professional Judgement in Health Care*. Elsevier, Edinburgh.

Fish, D. & Coles, C. (2005) *Medical Education: Developing a Curriculum for Practice*. Open University Press, Maidenhead.

Fish, D. & Twinn, S. (1997) *Quality Clinical Supervision in the Health Care Professions*. Reed, Oxford.

Fish, D., Twinn, S. & Purr, B. (1991) *Promoting Reflection: Improving the Supervision of Practice in Health Visiting and Initial Teacher Training*. West London Institute, London.

Freire, P. (1973) *Developing Critical Thinkers. Education as the Practice of Freedom in Education for Critical Consciousness*. Continuum, New York, NY.

Gibbs, G. (1988) *Learning by Doing: A Guide to Teaching and Learning Methods*. Further Education Unit, Oxford.

Gould, N. & Taylor, I. (1996) *Reflective Learning for Social Work*. Arena, Aldershot.

Greenwood, J. (1998) The role of reflection in single and double loop learning. *Journal of Advanced Nursing*. **27**, 1048–1053.

Habermas, J. (1974) *Theory and Practice*. Heinemann, London.

Horowitz, M.J. (1978) *Image Formation and Cognition*. Prentice Hall, New York, NY.

Johns, C. (1994) Nuances of reflection. *Journal of Clinical Nursing*. **3**, 71–75.

Johns, C. (2000) *Becoming a Reflective Practitioner*. Blackwell Science, Oxford.

Johns, C. (2002) *Guided Reflection. Advancing Practice*. Blackwell Science, Oxford.

Kelly, J. (1994) On reflection. *Practice Nurse*. **1** (14), 188–192.

Kemmis, S. (1985) Action research and the politics of reflection. In: *Reflection: Turning Experience into Learning* (eds D. Boud, R. Keogh & R. Walker). Kogan Page, London.

Knowles, M.S., Holton, H. & Swanson, R.A. (2005) *The Adult Learner*. Elsevier, Oxford.

Kolb, D.A. (1984) *Experiential Learning*. Prentice Hall, Upper Saddle River, NJ.

Mason, L. (1999) A cooperative inquiry study to identify strategies for group supervision in occupational therapy fieldwork placements. *Occupational Therapy International*. **6** (3), 224–242.

Mattingly, C. (1991) What is clinical reasoning? *American Journal of Occupational Therapy*. **45** (7), 979–986.

McGill, I. & Beatty, L. (1993) *Action Learning: A Practitioner's Guide*. Kogan Page, London.

Mezirow, J. (1981) A critical theory of adult learning and education. *Adult Education*. **32** (1), 3–24.

Moon, J. (1999) *Reflection in learning and professional development*. Kogan Page, London.

Nystrand, M. (1977) *Language as a Way of Knowing*, pp. 95–104. Ontario Institute for Studies in Education, Toronto.

Paterson, B.L. (1995) Developing and maintaining reflection in clinical journals. *Nurse Education Today*. **15** (6), 211–220.

Polyani, M. (1967) *Tacit Knowing*. Routledge and Kegan Paul, London.

Richardson, G. & Maltby, H. (1995) Reflection-on-practice: enhancing student learning. *Journal of Advanced Nursing*. **22** (6), 135–142.

Saylor, C. (1990) Reflection and professional education: arts, science and competency. *Nurse Educator*. **15** (2), 5–42.

Schell, B. & Cervero, R. (1993) Clinical reasoning in occupational therapy: an integrative review. *American Journal of Occupational Therapy*. **47** (7), 605–610.

Schön, D.A. (1983) *The Reflective Practitioner*. Arena, Aldershot.

Schön, D.A. (1987) *Educating the Reflective Practitioner*. Jossey Bass, San Francisco, CA.

Strong, J., Gilbert, J., Cassidy, S. & Bennett, S. (1995) Expert clinicians and students' views on clinical reasoning in occupational therapy. *British Journal of Occupational Therapy*. **58**, 119–123.

Taylor, M.C. (2000) *Evidence - Based Practice for Occupational Therapists*. Blackwell, Oxford.

Unsworth, C.A. (2004) Clinical reasoning: how do pragmatic reasoning, worldview and client centredness fit? *British Journal of Occupational Therapy*. **67** (1), 10–19.

Van Manen, M. (1977) Linking ways of knowing with ways of being practical. *Curriculum Inquiry*. **6** (3), 205–222.

9: A reflexive model for problem-based learning

Steven W. Whitcombe and Teena J. Clouston

Introduction

The previous chapter discussed reflection and its influences on problem-based learning (PBL) curricula. Here, we intend to focus on the tool of reflexivity and present a model that can enable this process for staff, students and organisations. For PBL to work effectively, there has to be congruence between this triad of elements. Organisational frames create cultural norms that can influence curricula and therefore how PBL programmes are exigent. On a more personal level, staff and students need to recognise their ontological position and juxtapose it with how PBL is realised within their unique organisational context. Our reflexive model is one tool to enable you to do this by challenging preconceptions and hidden disjunctures to foster cultural fit and personal harmony with PBL philosophy and practice, as PBL in any one setting is a co-produced phenomenon, constructed by individual meaning and cultural forms and identities.

PBL has been discussed elsewhere in this book. Consequently, we will not define it here. However, we do intend to bring together some of the main requirements and tools of PBL in terms of its construction, specifically those relevant to being a tutor facilitator and student-directed learner. First, we intend to clarify the meanings and purpose of reflexivity and contextualise its use in the model.

Reflexivity

Reflexivity can be defined as a dynamic process of positionality and personal reflection. Positionality can be understood in two ways. In the first sense, the self is seen as part of the social environment in which it is situated. It is, therefore, both familiar with and subsumed by that social frame (Goffman, 1974, 1981). Reflexivity in this sense challenges us to raise unconscious thoughts and behaviour to conscious awareness; to examine our own familiarity with and taken-for-granted approaches to everyday life at individual, organisational and societal life. In the second sense, positionality refers to your constructed identity in respect of socially defined markers such as age, gender, class, sexuality, culture and ethnicity. Reflection is the ability to challenge biases, prejudices, values and life experiences that shape how you view a particular phenomenon. Through reflexivity, biases and assumptions made manifest through reflection can be positioned into your personal life narrative. When understood in this way, reflexivity is a tool to illuminate and question both the what and the why of your unique perception of the life-world (Schutz, 1972). Finlay (2002) points out that social researchers have used the concept of reflexivity in different ways, including for example 'confessional tales' where researchers describe their study experiences, or as a way of examining their personal and social position in relation to a research project or used reflexivity as a method of critical reflection to monitor and self-audit the research process.

For our purposes, the intention of the model is to use reflexivity as a tool to examine both personal position – assumptions and values with regard to the subject matter – and the context in which the PBL will take place. Personal reflexivity involves acknowledging our own cultural and social values as well as our biases and assumptions – specifically, the views and assumptions we hold about PBL and the pre-existing knowledge we have in relation to this and traditional teaching forms about PBL. The methodological use of reflexivity will involve the need for a self-scrutinising approach to our role and assumptions in PBL.

The reflexive model

The model consists of the three elements we conceive as integral to PBL, that is the individual, the pedagogy of PBL and the organisation which together enables the self-reflexive project. This model builds on an earlier published version (Clouston & Whitcombe, 2005) and condenses our previous thoughts from a quintuple to a triadic form. The three elements represent factors, opportunities and challenges that interact synergically to influence the process and experience of PBL for all concerned. These can be summarised as below.

The individual and the self-reflexive project

Chapter 3 of this book examined the concept of 'readiness' for PBL and in doing so, it was posited that cognitive dissonance could be a negative or positive influence on the individual's engagement with PBL. Central to the model therefore, is the self-analysis of how 'ready' the individual is for the pedagogy, that is the educational approach of PBL and the dissonance that may be encountered through the experience of being a student of PBL or a facilitator on a PBL programme.

Atherton (2003) states that cognitive dissonance is a psychological phenomenon which refers to the discomfort felt at a discrepancy between what you already know or believe, and new information or interpretation. It therefore occurs when there is a need to accommodate new ideas, and it may be necessary for this to develop so that we can become 'open' to them. Both De Grave *et al.* (1998) and Neighbour (1992) suggest further, that dissonance can cause an intellectual wedge between current beliefs and reality and can cause resistance to learning.

Arguably, PBL adheres to a 'constructivist' view of learning which upholds the idea that individuals use and create knowledge in different ways, depending on their unique experiences (Hendry *et al.*, 1999). Within the espoused philosophy of PBL therefore, knowledge is viewed in a relativist (all answers are equally valued) rather than an absolute (single truth) manner.

The philosophical assumptions underpinning PBL support the constructivist position by encouraging the student or facilitator to explore multiple truths or multiple realities when addressing problem or case scenarios, opposing the belief that there is an absolute truth and therefore always a right or wrong answer to be found. If the ontological view that is held is one where knowledge is absolute then there will be difficulties in accepting the philosophy and application of PBL. As an individual student or tutor, this fundamental concept of congruence with the philosophical stance of knowledge has to be recognised and dissonance challenged if they are to be congruent with PBL philosophy. As this can be subliminal or unconscious, there may be a need to bring this to conscious thought and gain congruence in thinking and philosophical approach to learning.

Whilst some research has considered adults' readiness to engage with learning and teaching in higher education and the factors that help or hinder this process such as students' academic skills (Lowe & Cook, 2003) or their access to social support (Castles, 2004), there appears to be no research that specifically addresses students' readiness to engage with PBL. However, a key factor in determining an individual's readiness to engage with higher education in general may be dependent upon learning style. Cust (1996) and Prosser and Trigwell (1999) argue that this is related to an individual's previous experience of learning, including what has worked well for them in the past, and what an individual expects in terms of learning style from any new course they wish to undertake. Unlike traditional content-specific courses, PBL programmes require student and tutor participants to synthesise knowledge and understanding from the outset and accommodate a cooperative, group approach to learning where traditional power and relationship structures are fundamentally changed. Thus, when individuals embark on a PBL programme, they may be unprepared for this way of working and utilise a superficial rather than deep approach to learning in accord with past experience and applied strategies. In order to overcome this challenge, participants need to achieve a state of readiness and preparedness for PBL.

Preparedness suggests a particular skill level or willingness to learn the skills necessary to participate in PBL groups. Hay (1997) and Olmesdahl and Manning (1999) allude that this can be achieved through training for example, in constructive feedback methods, facilitation skills and communication strategies.

Haith-Cooper (2000) however, notes that no amount of training could change philosophical beliefs unless the individual is ready to do so. This state of readiness includes the ability to accept the role of adult learner and self-directed learning, to have trust in your own decisions and others, that is, confidence in peer knowledge and being self-supportive. Readiness also includes readiness to learn, to practice and develop new skills and willingness to overcome barriers to learning in different ways. In this respect, it seems that an individual's readiness to engage in PBL is closely linked to the concept of congruence. The key to success in PBL is that the participants in a learning environment are cognisant with and accepting enough of the principles to enable the effectiveness of the process. This may require an exploration of and a fundamental change in personal mindset (Kwan, 2000).

With this in mind, Johnson and Tinning (2001) propose that through reflective practice, PBL participants can challenge discrepancies between espoused theories and practice and therefore develop a higher level of self-awareness. Self-evaluation is a requisite skill in PBL but its use is framed by the degree of honesty and openness applied to critically exploring one's own fundamental beliefs and assumptions regarding learning (Hay, 1995). Therefore, to truly benefit from reflection and evaluation, a deep and personal level of reflexive analysis is required.

Reflexivity and the pedagogy of PBL

PBL as an educational approach concentrates on learning as opposed to teaching *per se*. Underpinned by constructivism, the pedagogy of PBL utilises methods of learning that encourage cooperation, integration and the critical application of knowledge. Therefore, group work is the cornerstone of PBL practice and since effective learning on a PBL programme requires small groups, the dynamics of the membership are influential on both learning experience and outcome. The enabling group dynamics include a shared sense of belonging, investment and commitment to the group, an ability to respond proactively, to meet group needs (Haith-Cooper, 2000) and development of the skills needed to solve problems individually and collectively.

As such, individuals need to be able to attain the skills to work in groups. Heron (1989) suggests that groups move through developmental stages including an initial stage of defensiveness whereby members' trust is low and anxiety high. As anxiety reduces, the group moves to a stage of authentic behaviour where trust is high, anxiety underpins growth and open communication takes place. At the final stage of closure, the group can reflect on their learning and generalise this to every day activity.

Savin-Baden (1997) discussed the concept of 'validated knowing' within PBL, where successful groups enabled synthesis of learning through feedback and support of individual learners and tutors. This function of learning was based on trust and feeling valued as a person within the group setting and the experience of being heard in the group. As group participants then, using your own experience, validating feedback and supporting others is an essential requirement to enrich learning.

Therefore, group work can be a positive learning experience but initially such dependency on this method of learning may be alien or incongruous with the individual student's or lecturer's previous ways of learning or teaching. Consequently, there is a need for individuals to be reflexive on how they function in the PBL group, their openness to group learning and the challenges and benefits that group work presents.

Reflexivity and the organisation

The implementation of PBL will vary according to the organisational setting and the perceived outcomes of different PBL programmes. Therefore, as individuals, we need to be reflexively conscious of the organisational and cultural factors that structure the pedagogy of PBL, that is, how PBL is constructed and delivered in your particular setting. Norms in the organisation can hinder or promote the development of the cultural change necessitated for PBL as there must be openness to difference and non-traditional teaching methods.

Little and Saucer (1991) argue that to enable a PBL-focused curriculum, requires both a proactive cultural and personal change. Whilst cultural and personal views can vary due to individual differences, the expectation and values of the staff group are inherent to the process of success. Thus transparency and empowerment within organisational domains is integral to effective implementation and outcome of PBL. This includes transparency of course expectations and requirements in terms of learning and identity of PBL philosophy. Where this is hidden, crystallisation and cohesion of an organisational form can be challenged.

The organisation has to nurture and accept the responsibility of the student to learn and the tutor to facilitate rather than deliver curricula; this requires a culture of trust, respect, non-judgementalism, honesty and participation (Rogers, 1983).

Learners can absorb the expectations and values of the organisation and if this seems to mirror a traditional, pedagogical way of teaching, students may adopt strategic methods of learning that can result in a limited use of problem solving or autonomous approaches (Entwistle & Ramsden, 1983; Savin-Baden, 1997). If clarity in the pedagogical or andragogical continuum is beyond the visible, or the known, then diametrical approaches to learning can develop.

Clear systems for communication at all levels within the PBL environment and wider organisation is central to effective PBL implementation. Open channels of communication enable empowerment and therefore, a person-centred culture (Rogers, 1983). Transparency around expected course outcomes to enable effective participation and learning should be a prerequisite of all higher education environments (Ramsden, 1992; Knight, 2002) and are essential components of participation and empowerment in PBL. The expectations of the learner may differ from the espoused outcomes of their educational programme. If this were to occur in PBL curricula, then the student's understanding of the key element of self-directed learning may differ from staff expectation. Moreover, competing rationalities, that is, opposing ideas, views and opinions can exist between the organisation (structure or culture) and PBL philosophy, on a micro scale between staff and student groups and also inter-staff and inter-student factions (Wilby & Clouston, 2003). Open forums for discussion can offer opportunity to challenge differences, exchange ideas and resolve potential disharmony.

Using the reflexive model

Figure 9.1 demonstrates how the model can be represented diagrammatically and how the three key elements interact with the need for the individual to be self-reflexive. It is the awareness and appreciation of these elements and how they coexist that we feel is central to a more insightful understanding of the nature of PBL and the individual's experience of it. Therefore, some key questions are offered in each of the elements as a guide to help both students and tutors reflect on the PBL process and their participation in it. In each section of the model, tutors and students can select pertinent questions in relation to their role as a PBL participant. The challenge for all individuals is to reflexively explore their own ideals, values and beliefs in regard to learning and teaching. The questions represent the findings from research undertaken that explored occupational therapy student's experiences of PBL (Clouston, 2005), an extensive literature review and the authors' own reflections of working on a PBL programme.

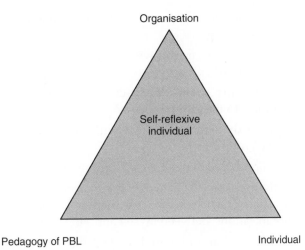

Figure 9.1 A reflexive model for problem-based learning.

Reflective questions of the individual

What is my view of learning – is this congruent with PBL philosophy?

Am I teacher or person centred?

What is my pedagogical/andragogical stance – what do I truly believe?

Am I doing what I say I'm doing?

Is my view of PBL congruent with the curriculum?

Is the organisational strategy congruent with PBL?

Am I or the group looking for right and wrong answers, for example, knowledge checking, finding facts, looking for single truths instead of multiple realities?

Is my thinking congruent with PBL?

Reflective questions of the pedagogy

How do I like to learn? Does my preferred learning style influence how I facilitate PBL groups?

How does my personality style influence group facilitation or participation? Am I over or under supportive, over or under challenging?

Am I ready to accept feedback from others about my facilitation style?

Am I prepared to vary my style according to the needs of the group?

Do I control the group or facilitate the group to run itself?

Am I ready to accept that individuals are responsible for their own and the group's learning?

Am I ready to facilitate self-directed learning?

Am I ready to relinquish the role of expert in subject knowledge?

Am I ready to accept tutors as facilitators rather than subject experts?

Am I ready to be honest about the limitations of my knowledge and understanding?

Am I ready to share this with other members of the group and the wider organisation?

Am I able to recognise the value of my contribution and the contribution of others to the group process?

Am I ready to recognise my learning needs to facilitate and participate in the group?

Am I prepared to meet these learning needs?

Am I prepared to challenge discrepancies between PBL-espoused theory and practice; between myself and other facilitators in the same organisations; between myself and PBL strategy?

Am I ready and prepared to challenge and change my own learning style in line with PBL philosophy?

Will I ever be ready to do so?

Reflective questions of the organisation

How are learning and teaching strategies communicated?

How are priorities for learning and teaching shared and to what extent are they valued by the organisation, staff, students and stakeholders?

What systems or opportunities (if any) are in place for me to discuss my role in the PBL environment?

Are there forums to facilitate and discuss ideas and developments in PBL for staff, students and others with opportunities to learn from each other?

How much time and investment is given to discussion of ideas?

If systems or strategies are not in place, how can I enable them?

How would I appraise my interpersonal communication skills? Am I able to communicate in groups?

Is there an organisational strategy on PBL?

What is my organisation's understanding, view or rationale on PBL?

Is there a cultural fit between organisational values and PBL theory?

To what extent does my personal interpretation of PBL reflect those of the organisation in which I work?

Do I feel constrained by the curriculum I have to deliver? Is it product or process orientated?

Is there transparency within curriculum delivery?

Is the curriculum sufficiently flexible to be delivered through a PBL approach?

Conclusion

In this chapter, we have presented a reflexive model of PBL that can be used by students and course tutors on PBL programmes to enhance the experience of this method of learning. The model considers three essential elements, the individual, the educational approach (pedagogy) and the organisation which interact with one another and enables consideration, reflection and evaluation individually and collectively as participants in PBL groups. We have offered a number of questions that can be used to promote the development of self-reflection or reflexivity within the context of PBL. We would argue further, that the model could also be used to develop PBL curricula and consider the organisational and cultural constraints or commonalities that will impinge on the PBL process.

References

Atherton, J.S. (2003) Learning and Teaching: Cognitive Dissonance [On-line], UK. Available at: file:///C:/Documents%20and%20Settings/Default/Desktop/Cognitive%20 dissonance.htm. Accessed on 10th July 2004.

Castles, J. (2004) Persistence and the adult learner: factors affecting persistence in open university students. *Active Learning in Higher Education*. **2** (5), 166–180.

Clouston, T.J. (2005) Facilitating tutorials in problem based learning; the students' per- spective. In: *Enhancing Teaching in Higher Education: New Approaches to Improving Student Learning* (eds P. Hartley, *et al.*), pp. 54–64. Routledge, London.

Clouston, T.J. & Whitcombe, S.W. (2005) An emergent person centred model for problem-based learning. *Journal of Further and Higher Education*. **29** (3), 265–279.

Cust, J. (1996) A relational view of learning: implications for nurse education. *Nurse Education Today*. **16**, 256–266.

De Grave, W.S., Dolmans, D.H.J.M. & van der Vleuten, C.P.M. (1998) Tutor intervention profile: reliability and validity. *Medical Education*. **32**, 262–268.

Entwistle, N. & Ramsden, P. (1983) *Understanding Student Learning*. Croom Helm, London.

Finlay, L. (2002) Outing the researcher. *Qualitative Health Research*. **12** (4), 531–545.

Goffman, E. (1974) *Frame Analysis: An Essay on the Organisation of Experience*. Harper Row, New York, NY.

Goffman, E. (1981) *Forms of Talk*. Basil Blackwell, Oxford.

Haith-Cooper, M. (2000) Problem-based learning within health professional education: what is the role of the lecturer? *Nurse Education Today*. **20**, 267–272.

Hay, J.A. (1995) Investigating the development of self evaluation skills in a problem based tutorial course. *Academic Medicine*. **70** (8), 733–735.

Hay, J.A. (1997) An investigation of a tutor evaluation scale for formative purposes in a problem based learning curriculum. *The American Journal of Occupational Therapy*. **51** (2), 140–143.

Hendry, G.D, Frommer, M. & Walker, R.A. (1999) Constructivism and problem-based learning. *Journal of Further and Higher Education*. **23** (3), 359–371.

Heron, J. (1989) *The Facilitators Handbook*. Kogan Page, London.

Johnson, A.K. & Tinnings, R.S. (2001) Meeting the challenge of problem based learning: developing the facilitators. *Nurse Education Today*. **21**, 161–169.

Knight, P.T. (2002) *Being a Teacher in Higher Education*. Open University Press, Buckingham.

Kwan, C.Y. (2000) What is problem based learning: it is magic, myth and mindset. *CDLT Brief*. **3**, 3. Available: http://www.cdtl.nus.edu.sg/brief/Pdf/v3n3.pdf. Accessed on 12th July 2004.

Little, S. & Saucer, C. (1991) Organisation and institutional impediments. In: *Problem Based Learning* (eds D. Boud & G. Feletti), pp. 88–95. Kogan Press, London.

Lowe, R. & Cook, A. (2003) Mind the gap: are students prepared for higher education? *Journal of Further and Higher Education*. **1** (27), 53–75.

Neighbour, R. (1992) *The Inner Apprentice*. Petroc Press, Plymouth.

Olmesdahl, P.J. & Manning, D.M. (1999) Impact of training on PBL facilitators. *Medical Education*. **33**, 753–755.

Prosser, N. & Trigwell, K. (1999) *Learning and teaching: the experience in higher education*. Society for Research in Higher Education and Open University Press, Buckingham.

Ramsden, P. (1992) *Learning to Teach in Higher Education*. Routledge, London.

Rogers, C. (1983) *Freedom to Learn for the 80's*. McMillan, New York, NY.

Savin-Baden, M. (1997) Problem based learning part 2: understanding learners stances. *British Journal of Occupational Therapy*. **60** (12), 531–536.

Schutz, A. (1972) *The Phenomenology of the Social World*, (trans G. Walsh & F. Lehnert). Heinemann Educational Books, London.

Wilby, P.K. & Clouston, T.J. (2003) Developing On-line Synthesis Groups to Support PBL. Conference Paper ENOTHE, Prague. Available at: http://www.enothe.hva.nl/meet/ac03/app_overhead_12.ppt.

10: Promoting creative thinking and innovative practice through the use of problem-based learning

Jill Riley and Ruth Matheson

Introduction

Today, students graduating from professional courses need to be prepared to meet the challenges of change and diversity in professional practice through an ability to solve problems and offer innovative solutions to complex situations. This chapter explores the links between creativity and problem-based learning (PBL) and challenges the reader to consider the need for promoting creative thinking leading to innovative practice. An exploration of the underlying theories of creativity highlights the attributes of a creative person who can respond adaptively, see beyond the immediate situation and redefine complex problems, important in a rapidly changing health and social care environment. The student-centred nature of PBL offers students opportunities to develop such attributes and become motivated and self-initiated learners with the ability to question and understand the complexity and diversity of everyday situations. This chapter will highlight the links between these theories and explore the challenge facing higher education in providing opportunities within the curriculum for students to develop their personal creative potential and utilise this in their chosen domain or field. Finally, findings from a qualitative longitudinal study, detailing PBL students' perceptions of factors that enhanced or inhibited their creativity within the PBL arena, will be identified and discussed.

The need for creativity and innovation in contemporary society

In contemporary Western and technological societies, individuals must engage with a fast and relentless pace of organisational change. Embracing this requires an ability to take on new ideas and come up with creative and innovative solutions to problems. Adaptability to change and creative problem-solving requires individuals to be able to constantly question their current perceptions and think creatively in order to address future challenges innovatively.

In preparing students for the future, higher education needs to focus not only on promoting academic knowledge, but providing the skills and basis for creative lateral thinking. This becomes particularly important in the education of emerging health and social care professionals who are required to come to the working environment with such qualities and attributes to meet professional standards.

Creativity is defined as

■ an ability to produce something new;
■ a novel and useful response to an open-ended task;
■ achieving something that is appropriate to a given situation;
■ seeing beyond the immediate situation and redefining problems;
■ intellectually engaging with materials;
■ a process of understanding self, seeing things differently, presenting novel ideas and conceptualisations.

(Kneller, 1966; Sternberg, 1988; Gardner, 1999)

The creative person has particular personal qualities and abilities, for instance

■ an ability to respond adaptively;
■ having high self-esteem;
■ good problem-solving skills;
■ being intrinsically rather than extrinsically motivated;
■ engage in activity primarily for its own sake.

Enhancing such qualities in students of different ages, gender, interests, abilities and intellect presents a challenge for higher education, particularly in a climate where widening access to courses means that students also come from diverse cultural, social and educational backgrounds. A further challenge is faced where programmes have a professional focus, for example the allied health professions, nursing or social work, where a professional or accreditation body demands particular curricula content as a requirement. This can make student choice and engagement in activities for their own sake problematic, thereby reducing intrinsic motivation. In health-care curricula for instance, there can be an emphasis on diagnosis-led outcomes which in turn drive the students towards predetermined solutions, rather than looking for a more creative and person-centred approach as central to the problem-solving process. Where learning outcomes focus on process rather than outcome however, students have more freedom to explore and respond adaptively, which promotes problem-solving skills and enhances their self-esteem.

A particular challenge then for health and social care programmes is how to enhance students' creative qualities and abilities whilst satisfying professional and organisational requirements, issues addressed in later sections of this chapter. In the first instance, in order to provide a context, we consider theories of creativity and the link between creativity and PBL.

Theories of creativity

Theories of creativity have been developed from different psychological perspectives: psychoanalytical, which are concerned with the expression of inner drives and conflict with the unconscious mind; behavioural, which considers creativity as a form of novel behaviour resulting from unusual environmental conditions; developmental, which is concerned with the importance of developmental stages and emphasises the need for psychometric testing, and creative cognition which emphasises human beings' capacity for creative thought (Kneller, 1966; Gardner, 1982; Runco, 1991; Gruber & Wallace, 1999). Here, we focus on a humanistic approach and a belief that creativity comes from an individual's openness and ability to engage with the world leading to self-fulfilment and self-actualisation (Rogers, 1961; Maslow, 1968). In addition, drawing on Csikszentmihalyi's (1996) view of creativity, we also take a systems approach, seeing the creative individual as interacting within a socio-cultural context and bringing creative ideas to a specific domain.

A humanistic approach to creativity

From a humanistic perspective, everyone has the potential to be creative; it is a process of self-actualisation (Maslow, 1968). We are all creative to a greater or lesser degree (Kneller, 1966). Creative individuals are generally described in the psychology literature as adaptable, flexible, open to new ideas, attracted to complexity and intrinsically motivated (Amabile, 1996; Collins & Amabile, 1999; Sternberg & Lubart, 1999). In other words, there can be different levels of creativity and, within higher education, it is important to take this into account and value, promote and foster creativity in all students. This is something that PBL, through a person-centred approach to learning and teaching, has the potential to achieve.

A systems approach to creativity

In higher educational environments, students usually learn about, develop and ultimately contribute to a particular subject area or domain. Within health and social care, this can include the knowledge base associated with a specific profession and the organisational systems in which the profession operates. Csikszentmihalyi (1996) points out that the domain has a culturally situated set of symbolic rules and procedures, which need to be internalised before individuals can make a creative contribution. Additionally, individuals need to be familiar with the field, that is; the specific area where creative contributions can impact, together with the requirements of the experts within it. Initially, students require access to the domain and opportunities to develop their cultural and educational capital (Chapter 11) through exposure to a rich educational environment (Csikszentmihalyi, 1996). In PBL, that environment includes the student group and facilitating tutor; their impact on students' creative development is discussed in later sections of this chapter.

Phases of creativity

The process of generating creative ideas involves moving through certain phases or steps. A traditional view of this is encapsulated in a classical analytical framework, originating from the work of Wallas (1926) and developed by Csikszentmihalyi (1996, p. 78). It comprises the following:

- Preparation: being immersed in problematic issues that arouse curiosity.
- Incubation: churning around ideas.
- Insight: the 'aha' moment when the ideas fit together.
- Evaluation: deciding if an idea is worth pursuing.
- Elaboration: putting it together and making it work.

The process is not linear and may go through many loops and iterations depending on the breadth and depth of issues explored (Csikszentmihalyi, 1996). In health and social care curricula for instance, problems and issues are contextual and the focus is not only on the individual who requires intervention, but incorporates their socio-cultural environment together with the organisation and profession. The domain therefore, is complex and the students' ability to internalise it and generate creative solutions to problems can depend on opportunities for them to engage in a creative process.

Link between creativity and PBL

It became evident to us as tutors with an interest in the theory of creativity, that there are close links between the problem-solving process utilised in PBL and the creative analytical framework.

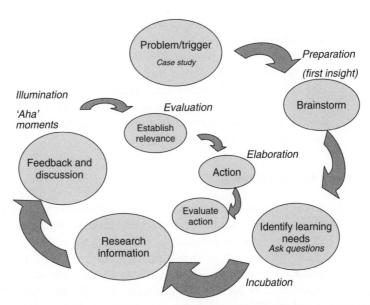

Figure 10.1 A problem-based learning (PBL) cycle (Riley & Matheson, 2005) linked to the creative analytical framework (Csikszentmihalyi, 1996). Key: the *grey ovals* and *arrows* represent a PBL cycle. The *italicised text* places the creative analytic framework in the PBL cycle.

Placing the creative process within our PBL cycle (Figure 10.1), indicated to us where students' creativity might be enhanced by the PBL process. Preparation is about being immersed in problematic issues that occur during the brainstorming stage; incubation, the churning around ideas, comes from the need to ask questions and identify issues; insight comes from the 'aha' moments when the ideas fit together following discussion and feedback; evaluation is concerned with deciding if ideas are worth pursuing by establishing their relevance. Finally, elaboration is about putting it all together and making it work, in other words taking action and evaluating that action.

There is also a perceptible link between the attributes of a creative person, highlighted in theories of creativity and those developed through PBL. The student-centred nature of PBL offers students opportunities to develop the creative attributes described above and become motivated and self-initiated learners with the ability to question and understand the complexity and diversity of everyday situations (Knowles, 1980; Barrows, 1994; Savin-Baden, 2000).

Having made the links, as tutors, between the attributes of the creative thinker and those developed through PBL, we felt that there was a need to explore the students' perceptions of the importance and development of these skills and whether or not these were enhanced or inhibited through the use of PBL. The following sections present the findings from a qualitative longitudinal study following one cohort of students through a 3-year occupational therapy degree programme, utilising focus groups to gather data. Students identified four key factors that enhanced or inhibited their creativity within the PBL curriculum: the learning environment, tutor facilitation, the presenting problem or trigger and opportunities to develop self-understanding. These will be discussed further, using the students' words (presented in italics) to emphasise salient points.

The learning environment

Creativity can be enhanced in an environment where students can freely exchange ideas, explore interests and there is opportunity for choice and discovery (Collins & Amabile, 1999; Nickerson, 1999). In order to foster creativity, the environment needs to be comfortable, safe, supportive and flexible enough for students to try out new ideas. For students, a major part of such an environment is their PBL group. The bond they develop within the group has a profound effect on their development of creative thinking; this can be compared with a therapeutic relationship where clients need a supportive environment in order to take risks and make changes (Schmid, 2004). As one student put it:

> I think it's just the bonding with your group, the whole getting to know people. I think you begin to trust people and not feel that an idea you might say, you might think's OK, but sometimes you're worried about other people's reaction maybe.

The students needed to build confidence and trust in each other in order to feel safe to try out new ideas. This happens over time and it was not until students are well established in the course that they feel able to confidently challenge each other:

> I suppose its trial and error through presenting and being in your group and feeling comfortable with people. You can take those skills with you then because you've learnt them in a positive way in stead of being punished or embarrassed in front of someone.

Johnson and Johnson (2006) propose that creative insights occur when group members have different viewpoints and come to the group with diverse information. Creativity is enhanced further when group members disagree and are able to challenge each others' ideas constructively (Paulus *et al.*, 2001). However, when the social environment is not supportive and group members become threatened, or pressured, creative thinking becomes stifled. This lack of group cohesion not only reduces creative thinking but also decreases motivation:

> if you're not getting on with your group then it's going to put a block on it . . . you don't feel you can really have a good discussion, cos people don't want to be there so you don't really have that free-thinking.

The challenge for educators here is how to enhance students' group working skills and promote group cohesion in order to allow creativity to flourish. The incubation stage of the problem-solving process particularly, demands persistence and potentially conflicting ideas can lead to frustration, tension and discomfort (Johnson & Johnson, 2006). This needs to be recognised by the group as a part of the process of formulating creative solutions. Adopting group rules may assist in eliminating the minor conflicts, but group members also need encouragement to analyse tensions and take responsibility for both their learning and behaviour within the group. Recognising individual differences and seeing these as an asset to promote diverse thinking might, for instance, be achieved through use of the reflective model discussed in Clouston and Whitcombe (2005).

In terms of the physical environment, the type of room, space and time to meet as a group also affect students' ability to develop creative thinking. The imposition of pre-arranged timetables, room booking systems and malfunctioning equipment often have a detrimental impact on the free-flow of ideas. Whilst recognising the reality of organisational constraints, educators need to highlight the importance of flexibility when planning PBL programmes.

Tutor facilitation that promotes the development of creative thinking

Tutor facilitation within PBL, because of its centrality to the process and development of student-centred learning, has been the topic of much debate. Facilitation in this instance is defined as:

> a goal orientated dynamic process in which participants work together in an atmosphere of genuine mutual respect, in order to learning through critical reflection.
>
> (Burrows 1997, p. 401)

However, this student-centred and participatory approach to facilitation may not always be put into practice. Drinan (1997) proposes that many teachers think they are facilitating students whilst in reality, they are conducting teacher-centred tutorials; others, according to Maudsley (1999, p. 657), are mistaking 'student-centred' for 'tutor-inactive'. The tutor's role in Dolmans *et al*. (2005) view, is to scaffold student learning by stimulating discussion, providing stimulus for elaboration, encouraging the integration of knowledge and promoting interaction between students. This is achieved through asking questions, seeking clarification and providing insights to enhance the application of knowledge.

The students in our study identified the type of questioning as crucial to the development of their creative thinking. Tutors who purely asked the students 'what do you think' without constructively stimulating elaboration induced panic because the students felt that they were being examined and had to provide the right answer:

Passive questioning which just throws the question straight back at you gets in the way ... panic ... paralyses thought.

Tutors need to encourage open thinking, initial insights and the incubation of ideas that then lead to a variety of possible solutions. If this is closed down too quickly, then the potential for creative thinking is lost and a standardised answer is given. The students felt that tutors who could provide an ideational context for the problem enhanced their creative thinking by providing them with a visual picture from which they could spiral off their ideas. Tutors opened up thinking when they could rephrase the problem, provide similar examples or different contexts to promote the flow of ideas.

Being prompted encourages thinking .... Clarifying .... Broadening .... A range of ways to tackle a question.

Students felt that tutors who could engage with them and become part of the group could motivate learning through role modelling and their own enthusiasm for the subject matter. Moust cited in Schmidt and Moust (1995) defines this as role congruence when the tutor is willing to be part of the group and a student among the students, developing an informal relationship and demonstrating a caring and interested approach.

a lot of lecturers are quite prepared to use their own self and their own experiences and they bring themselves to the session, whereas others are quite stuck in the philosophy of PBL and it seems to put up a barrier

Tutors who had ownership of the course and knowledge of the subject matter were felt to be better placed to facilitate the group and generate creative solutions. Whereas tutors who 'dipped in' for the odd case study, lacked ownership, or had a poor knowledge of the curriculum as a whole, were considered to be less able to provide a context for creative thinking. As a consequence, students felt a lack confidence in their use of self and saw the facilitator's role as very passive. According to Moust, effective tutors demonstrate cognitive congruence, that is, an ability to express themselves in a language understandable by the students. Moust argues that this can only be achieved if tutors have a relevant knowledge base, and lines of enquiry and reasoning cannot be adequately followed without this knowledge ...

they think they can't bring anything to the session of themselves and I think that's when you get into the scenario of every question is bounced back at you rather than giving an example and a direction

The students valued tutor input that was meaningful and related to the 'real world' rather than directing students towards a hidden agenda. Transparency in the process and product is needed so that students feel that information is not being actively withheld and that learning becomes a game of hide and seek. Tutors that facilitate an environment of openness and trust within the group and encourage group evaluation on a regular basis, allowing for both peer and tutor review, were recognised as creating an environment where creative thought flourished, findings reiterated by Clouston (2004). The students felt this openness promoted effective group processes which ultimately impact on individual's confidence to offer alternative ideas.

> I think you begin to trust . . . . As you go through the course I think you can be more open and think more broadly within your group.

According to Dolmans *et al.* (2005), the tutor's task is concerned with keeping the learning process going, probing students' knowledge and ensuring that they are all involved in the process. In addition, tutors must monitor individual student's progress together with the challenge of the problem. Students require encouragement to think laterally in the first instance, but if, as one student put it:

> . . . it goes too broad that you just get totally lost . . . . You need to be brought back to the subject.

Therefore, tutors may need to take action and bring students back to the problem and harness their creativity to find a solution, in other words, the tutor's role is also concerned with maintaining a focus (Clouston, 2005).

Triggers that enhance creative problem-solving

Modern insights into learning suggest that 'learning always takes place within a context' (Dolmans *et al.*, 2005, p. 733) and one of the benefits of PBL is that it contextualises learning, relating it to the real world rather than being driven by curriculum content which is then translated into practice. If students are given the opportunity to look at problems in multiple contexts then, according to Ertmer and Newby (1993), they can develop their ability to transfer knowledge from one situation to another and this, in turn, promotes flexible and creative thinking.

For this to happen, the presenting problem requires a context that is firmly rooted in real life. Students felt that they need to be able to visualise the problem and picture the situation. Such visualisation is enhanced by the tutors' ability to paint a picture to tell a story using examples from their own experience:

> I think quite imaginatively, so I think in pictures . . . . When you put it into context it can clarify ideas.

This, in turn, facilitates students' development of appropriate and novel solutions to the problem. Embedding knowledge in prior experience provides security for students to expand their ideas and transfer knowledge into other situations. Tutors who could also prompt students into providing their own context could enhance creative thinking yet further:

> I think when you're asked to think of a place where you maybe have experienced something then you tend to think about it and relate it to a situation.

The type of problem or trigger is a major factor in enhancing or hindering creative problem-solving. Lloyd-Jones *et al.* (1998) state that the type of problem presented to students has a significant impact on the outcome and highlight that two styles of triggers are predominantly in use: firstly, an 'ill defined problem' (p. 492) and secondly, the narrative trigger, that lays a set of well-defined clues.

The use of narrative-type case studies where students are given detailed content can lead students to develop a word-spotting technique in an attempt to quickly identify the perceived solution to the problem. In a similar way to following the bread crumb trail in the story of Hansel and Gretel to lead them out of the forest, the case study can inadvertently lead students to a perceived right answer. This content-driven approach pushes the student to find textbook solutions, limiting the discussion with the emphasis on outcome rather than the learning process. Consequently, the process then becomes tutor-led (Lloyd-Jones *et al.* 1998).

However, this can be altered to enhance creativity. Whilst recognising the need for content, the ability to visualise the problem is key. The use of pictures, story boards, cartoons, video clips and experiential learning are potential triggers that can generate creative thinking. Being presented with cases from a variety of perspectives helps students to challenge previous assumptions and stimulates the transfer of knowledge (Dolmans *et al.*, 2005), thus providing them with the opportunity to develop novel solutions.

From our study, one of the experiences that the students valued most in promoting their creative thinking was the use of role-play actors. This provides them with the opportunity to explore far beyond the paper case study, and, through a real-life presentation, arrive at realistic goals that are truly person-centred.

> And I think that's why it was so useful having the actors come in ... then you did have the person to sit down with and ask him or her things.

The development of such opportunities is one of the key challenges in PBL curriculum design. Problems should call upon the students' prior knowledge, allowing them to deconstruct it, incorporate new ideas, and generate discussion before finally reconstructing their learning to find a solution (Dolmans *et al.*, 2005). It is this opportunity for incubation of ideas through discussion and evaluation that allows the students to develop as creative problem solvers.

Promoting students' self-understanding

In order to become self-motivated and self-initiated learners with an ability to develop creative attributes, students require self-understanding and the opportunity for personal growth and self-actualisation (Rogers, 1961). In the context of PBL, this can come from a freedom to explore ideas, develop skills, establish trust, examine feelings and be able to reflect on those feelings. The students who took part in the study felt that they needed sufficient supported opportunities to develop their creative skills and ideas, for instance, through practical and experiential alongside other learning opportunities as a part of the PBL process. As one student put it:

> .. you get to sort of, I don't know, learn about yourself and use that . . . knowing 'what makes you tick'.

Experiential learning as an active form of learning (Burnard, 1991) can open up opportunities for the development of creative ideas and skills. Creativity is enhanced through opportunities for choice and discovery (Nickerson, 1999) and tutors need to encourage exploration and support students in trying out different ways of developing creative ideas and skills. For one student, it is about

> . . . maybe just getting a taste, rather than being able to be actually good at something, just having tried it to know what its about and not being worried about trying something new . . .

This is indeed an important part of the process and additionally, for students on health and social care courses, experiential learning can assist them in developing the skills they need for practice within their chosen domain, but to be creative within it, students need to internalise the rules of that domain (Csikszentmihalyi, 1996). This requires them to practice and hone skills and recognise their own strengths and limitations through a process of self-understanding.

An important aspect of understanding oneself, particularly in the context of PBL, which relies on group work, is learning about each other

> 'I think that having to trust people as well . .' and 'think differently'

For Csikszentmihalyi (1996), an awareness and appreciation of others' contributions to the domain puts one's own creativity into perspective. This requires mutual trust together with an ability to examine and reflect on one's own feelings and the attributes of creative experiences (Kolb, 1984) in order to make sense of them and put them in context. For this to happen, students need time and space for critical reflection in a supportive learning environment and an organisational climate where this is valued (Wisdom, 2006).

Conclusion

Our findings and discussion identify the links between the creative analytical framework and the PBL learning cycle. PBL is clearly a useful tool, given the right conditions, for the enhancement of creative thinking. For this to happen however, a number of prerequisites need to be addressed. In the first place, the learning environment must provide a sense of security to encourage students to challenge and question; developing students' readiness to engage in PBL and accept responsibility for individual and group learning is a fundamental part of the process. The reflective model proposed by Clouston and Whitcombe (2005) takes this further in that it challenges both the learner and educator to recognising the value of the group through a person-centred approach.

The need for clear ownership of the curriculum and a shared understanding of the nature of tutor facilitation is essential for the promotion of creative thinking. This places a responsibility on higher education establishments to provide continuing professional development opportunities to help staff acquire skills in facilitation that balance challenge with reinforcement, encourage questioning and provide a context from which students can generate ideas. New members of staff require time to understand the curriculum and develop confidence in their abilities to be able to create opportunities that foster students' creative thinking. It is a tutor's ability to promote open thinking and visualisation of practice, through the use of imaginative trigger material that appears to have the most impact on students being able to think outside the box. This has implications for curriculum design in that time and resources are needed to produce imaginative, relevant and appropriate problems or triggers. It also raises questions regarding the focus of staff development systems such as peer review, modelling, workshops and personal development planning.

In addition, experiential learning within the PBL provides opportunities for students to develop confidence to try out new ideas, acquire skills and ultimately gain a better understanding of self – qualities that are inherent in creative individuals. Within the constantly changing environment of health and social care, such qualities are essential to be able to gain an understanding of the complex nature of individuals' problems and seek creative solutions that meet their needs.

References

Amabile, T. (1996) *Creativity in Context*. WestView Press, Boulder, CO.

Barrows, H.S. (1994) *Problem-Based Learning Applied to Medical Education*. Southern Illinois School of Medicine, Springfield, IL.

Burnard, P. (1991) *Experiential Learning in Action*. Avebury, Aldershot.

Burrows, D.E. (1997) Facilitation: A concept analysis. *Journal of Advanced Nursing*. **25**, 396–404.

Clouston, T.J. (2005) Facilitating tutorials in problem-based learning. In: *Enhancing Teaching in Higher Education* (eds P. Hartley, A. Woods & M. Pill), pp. 48–58. Routledge, Oxford.

Clouston, T.J. & Whitcombe, S. (2005) An emerging person centred model for problem-based learning. *Journal of Further and Higher Education.* **29** (3), 265–275.

Collins, M. & Amabile, T. (1999) Motivation and creativity. In: *The Handbook of Creativity* (eds R. Sternberg), pp. 297–313. Cambridge University Press, Cambridge.

Csikszentmihalyi, M. (1996) *Creativity: Flow and the Psychology of Discovery and Invention.* HarperCollins, New York, NY.

Dolmans, D., De Grave, W., Wolfhagen, I. & van der Vleuten, C. (2005) Problem-based learning: future challenges for educational practice and research. *Medical Education.* **39**, 732–741.

Drinan, J. (1997) The limits of problem-based learning. In: *The Challenge of Problem-Based Learning* (eds D. Boud & G. Feletti), 2nd edn. pp. 333–339. Kogan Page, London.

Ertmer, P.A. & Newby, T.J. (1993) Behaviourism, cognitivism, constructivism: comparing critical features from an instructional design perspective. *Perform Improve Q.* **6** (4), 50–72.

Gardner, H. (1982) *Art, Mind and Brain: A Cognitive Approach to Creativity.* Basic Books, New York, NY.

Gardner, H. (1999) *Intelligence Reframed: Multiple Intelligences for the 21st Century.* Basic Books, New York, NY.

Gruber, H. & Wallace, D. (1999) The case study method and evolving systems approach for understanding unique creative people at work. In: *The Handbook of Creativity* (eds R. Sternberg), pp. 93–116. Cambridge University Press, Cambridge.

Johnson, D. & Johnson, F. (2006) *Joining Together, Group Theory and Group Skills,* 9th edn. Allyn and Bacon, Boston, MA.

Kneller, G. (1966) *The Art and Science of Creativity.* Rinehart, New York, NY.

Knowles, M. (1980) *The Modern Practice of Education: From Pedagogy to Andragogy.* Associated Press, Chicago, IL.

Kolb, D. (1984) *Experiential Learning Experience as the Source of Learning and Development.* Prentice Hall, Upper Saddle River, NJ.

Lloyd-Jones, G., Margetson, D. & Bligh, J. (1998) Problem-based learning: a coat of many colours. *Medical Education.* **32**, 402–494.

Maslow, A. (1968) *Toward a Psychology of Being.* John Wiley & Sons, New York, NY.

Maudsley, G. (1999) Roles and responsibilities of the problem based learning tutor in the undergraduate medical curriculum. *British Medical Journal.* **3** (18), 657–661.

Nickerson, R. (1999) Enhancing creativity. In: *The Handbook of Creativity* (eds R. Sternberg), pp. 392–431. Cambridge University Press, Cambridge.

Paulus, P.B., Larey, T.S. & Dzindolet, M.T. (2001) Creativity in groups and teams. In: *Groups at Work: Theory and Research* (eds M.E. Turner), pp. 319–338. Lawrence Erlbaum, Mahwah, NJ.

Riley, J. & Matheson, R. (2005) *Enhancing Students' Creativity Through Problem-Based Learning: A Challenge for Curriculum Design.* Paper given at International Conference on Problem-based Llearning, Lahti, Finland, June 2005.

Rogers, C. (1961) *On Becoming a Person: A Therapists' View of Psychotherapy*. Constable and Company, London.

Runco, M. (1991) *Divergent Thinking*. Ablex Publishing Co., Norwood, NJ.

Savin-Baden, M. (2000) *Problem-Based Learning in Higher Education: Untold Stories*. Open University Press, Buckingham.

Schmid, T. (2004) Meanings of creativity within occupational therapy practice. *Australian Occupational Therapy Journal*. **51** (2), 80–88.

Schmidt, H. & Moust, J. (1995) What makes a tutor effective? A structural-equations modelling approach to learning in problem-based curricular. *Academic Medicine*. **70** (8), 708–714.

Sternberg, R. (1988) *The Nature of Creativity*. Cambridge University Press, Cambridge.

Sternberg, R. & Lubart, T. (1999) The concept of creativity: prospects and paradigms. In: *The Handbook of Creativity* (eds R. Sternberg), pp. 3–16. Cambridge University Press, Cambridge.

Wallas, G. (1926) *The Art of Thought*. Watts and Co., London.

Wisdom, J. (2006) Developing higher education teachers to teach creatively. In: *Developing Creativity in Higher Education: An Imaginative Curriculum* (eds N. Jackson, N. Oliver, M. Shaw & J. Wisdom). Routledge, London.

11: Problem-based learning and the development of capital

Jill Riley and Steven W. Whitcombe

Introduction

Problem-based learning (PBL) is a constructive, interactive and student-centred form of learning that, as a process, is dependent upon the meaningful contributions of students and tutors. Typically in PBL courses, students of different ages, gender, socio-cultural and educational backgrounds come together in small groups with a facilitating tutor to share knowledge, learn from each other and work together to explore a diverse range of complex problems pertinent to their chosen area of study. Individual students and tutors bring to the PBL process both human capital in the form of different skills and abilities facilitated through previous education and training and cultural capital coming from traditional practices, educational and shared values.

This chapter explores how human and cultural capital continues to be developed by individuals in a PBL context and how it is utilised by the group for the creation of social capital. Through an exploration of the different forms of capital, drawing on the work of Bourdieu, Coleman, Putman and others, we will discuss how PBL groups can develop mutual trust and reciprocity, promoting the sharing of ideas and skills – the foundations of social capital. Through networking and sharing knowledge with other students, academics, professionals and others outside the group, such capital is developed for the common good. In addition, the authors explore how PBL can equip students to continually develop human and cultural capital through lifelong learning, and become responsible and active members of a profession that can contribute to the development of social capital for the benefit of society.

Forms of capital

Human and cultural capital are developed and processed by individuals whereas social capital is inherent in the structure of relations between people (Coleman, 1988; Fine & Green, 2000). Human capital is created by changes in the individual, bringing about skills and capabilities facilitated through education and training; it is embodied in an individual's skills and knowledge (Coleman, 1988; Becker, 1993). Cultural capital concerns 'the customs of public behaviour and the content of shared values' (Grew, 2001, p. 69). Like human capital, cultural capital is integral to the individual and requires the investment of time. It can be objectified in the form of 'cultural goods' such as works of art, books or instruments and institutionalised in the form of academic qualifications (Bourdieu, 1986, p. 47). Social capital, on the other hand, is less tangible, existing in social connections.

Human, cultural and social capital can be seen as complementary (Coleman, 1994; Grew, 2001). Individual students accrue human and cultural capital through education, personal backgrounds and life experiences, which are socio-culturally contextual. Individual skills and competencies, acquired and developed through formal and informal education, training and lifelong learning, constitute human capital whereas the development of professional knowledge in a cultural health and social care context and objectified in the form of a professional qualification constitutes cultural capital (Bourdieu, 1986; Grew, 2001). These forms of capital are personal to the individual and evolve over a lifetime (Fine & Green, 2001). They also constitute a rich resource for the individual to draw on when networking with others.

Social capital, then, refers to 'networks of social connection', in other words, 'doing with' others (Putman, 2000, p. 116). Being a health or social care professional often involves working in teams. PBL, with its emphasis on group working, helps students to learn the skills of team working such as shared decision making. Through working with others, students develop a specific, shared value system which is pertinent to their chosen profession. It is this value system or set of norms, which is shared amongst group members, permitting them to work together for common ends that defines social capital (Fukuyama, 1999). Before discussing the possible connection between PBL and the building of capital, it is necessary in the first instance to explore the significance of human and social capital for modern western societies such as the United Kingdom.

Forms of capital, globalising economies and higher education

Arguably, the accumulation of human, cultural and social capital and its acquired benefits take on particular significance for not only health professionals but also individuals in Western economies like the United Kingdom that are in the process of change. Worldwide influences as a consequence of globalisation are altering both how we live our lives and the forms of capital we require in order to adapt to a new social and economic order.

The simplest use of the term 'globalisation' encapsulates the notion that human beings are increasingly living in a shrinking world, one of global integration with an erosion of geographical borders due to technological advancements and expanding social, cultural and economic activity (Held & McGrew, 2000). Recent advancements (within the last 20 years) in telecommunication systems and electronic networks now offer a timeless medium of cultural exchange between societies and individuals throughout the world.

The outcomes of globalisation have consequences for individuals, and according to Beck (2001), modern society now equates to living in a risk society. For Beck, before globalisation, industrialised societies such as the United Kingdom were generally stable in terms of social structure, employment was plentiful and people tended to live 'standard biographies' (Beck, 2001, p. 166). In this regard, life patterns were often linear, and individuals were generally rooted in geography as were the firms/companies who employed them. Therefore, individuals tended to be meshed in strong social networks and traditional ways of living.

Since globalisation, life for people in modern society, or the 'second modernity' (Beck, 1999, p. 10), is demarcated through the process of 'elective biographies' and 'risk biographies' (Beck, 2001, p. 166). The changing nature of work has made employment less predicable for the individual and people are now much more 'on their own'. Correspondingly, social groups have become more fragmented, and conventional social bonds from which earlier generations might have taken support are replaced with less stable, ephemeral social networks.

Beck (2001) maintains that globalisation creates more options for people, but also more uncertainty and more risk, whilst Giddens (1998) points out that humans have always faced risk, for example, risk from natural disasters such as flooding; what is new is this 'manufactured' risk that arises out of a less economically ordered modern society.

Throughout the world and particularly in post-industrial societies such as the United Kingdom, changing economies are impacting on systems of higher education in terms of the purpose of universities. Societies in the 'second modernity' are beginning to generate national educational policies and directives in response to the new global economy (Hargreaves, 2003). In order to compete in a globalised world, modern societies are embracing the knowledge economy that is recognising that since the late twentieth century onwards, knowledge and information rather than fixed commodities such as land and localised work forces will become the main source of their wealth (Pruett & Schwellenbach, 2004). An example of this can be seen in a United Kingdom Government 1998 White Paper, *Our Competitive Future: Building the Knowledge Driven Economy*, which states that in the global economy, British businesses need to exploit distinctive capabilities which 'are not raw materials, land or access to cheap labour ... they must be knowledge, skills and creativity' (Department of Trade and Industry, 1998, p. 2).

In the United Kingdom, the Dearing (1997) review of higher education called for a new vision of learning and teaching in the university sector and one which is inclusive to all members of society. National governments are driving their universities/higher education institutions to respond to the knowledge economy in a variety of ways, including, for example, expanding their higher education provision to equip more people with the skills and knowledge necessary to embrace the knowledge economy, and consequently requiring their universities to place stronger emphasis on the development of lifelong learning skills and human capital (Field, 2000; Hargreaves, 2003).

In Britain, the expansion of student numbers, that is 'massification' (Henkel, 2000) in response to the knowledge economy has meant that the university has become more diverse in terms of its population, which in turn widens the opportunity to generate social capital. At the same time, however, the expansion of student numbers leads to a higher qualified workforce and, in essence, creates credential inflation (Brown, 1997). Therefore, in a market where up to 50% of the potential workforce are educated to degree level, the possession of rich forms of human and social capital can equip the individual with significant competitive advantage. The next section will consider how PBL and its espoused purpose correlates with the requirements of the 'knowledge economy'.

Knowledge economy and problem-based learning

PBL is an approach to learning that is intended to foster skills of critical analysis, self-evaluation and interpersonal communication. Epistemologically, PBL is underpinned by the idea that knowledge is not fixed and stable but, on the contrary, is fluid, transient and in many cases, obsolescent. Consequently, PBL curricula emphasise the contextual application of knowledge and learning outcomes that reflect learning as a process rather than the acquisition of facts.

By its very nature, PBL goes some way to enabling students develop the meta-cognitive and interactive skills that are necessary to adapt to a constantly changing world. Margetson (1994) posits that through its use of group work and cooperative problem solving, PBL helps students to acquire the capabilities to flourish in not just a changing world but more specifically, an increasingly pluralistic health and social care system. Thus, PBL offers the skills of critical contestability (Savin-Baden, 2003) that encourage lifelong learning and adaptability for the health/social care practitioner's career. Central to the development of lifelong learning skills such as reflection, critical reasoning and problem resolution addressed through PBL is the building of capital through the *process* of learning. What will follow are some examples of how the educational approach of PBL enables individuals to construct both social and human capital. In practice, these different forms of capital are constructed concurrently and are not therefore mutually exclusive. However, for the purposes of analysis, they will be considered separately. In the first instance, the development of social capital will be considered through the use of group work which is integral to PBL. Secondly, the development of human capital will be illustrated through a closer inspection of the life skills students attain through the PBL process.

Social capital, group work and PBL

There is empirical evidence that suggests that social capital in the form of stable social networks can promote the cognitive and social development of children (Field, 2005). For example, Coleman (1988) found that school children's academic performance was influenced positively by the existence of community ties between parents, teachers, neighbours and the church.

There is less direct research evidence to link social capital and adult learning. However, the process of group working within PBL suggests that social capital may contribute significantly to students' learning.

PBL is a collaborative form of learning in which problem resolution is dependent upon students working together and pooling resources both within and outside of the academic environment. Therefore, the life experience, skills and knowledge each individual brings to the PBL group and crucially shares with the group creates the social capital from which they can all benefit. Learning through PBL is thus co-constructed through the variegated experiences of students (and facilitators) and their different social backgrounds, for example, in respect of gender, age, class, ethnic origin and so on. Through the process of social networking and disclosure of experience, students not only learn *about* each other but *from* each other and furthermore, they may begin to redefine their pre-existing world view, that is their sense of 'habitus' (Bourdieu, 1990). However, self disclosure and cooperative learning require trust, which is fundamental to the notion of social capital (Coleman, 1994; Putman, 2000). As Fukuyama (1999, p. 16) argues, trust is 'like a lubricant that makes the running of any group or organisation more efficient'.

Close ties and strong levels of trust promote the sharing of information, ideas and skills (Field *et al.*, 2000) in a reciprocal way. Individuals must be prepared to make resources available to each other on concessionary terms and may reciprocate by paying debts in the course of time (Portes, 1998). The ability to do something for someone without any immediate return forms the 'touchstone' of social capital (Putman, 2000, p. 134).

From the perspective of PBL, research within health care has demonstrated the importance of group trust in enabling learning (e.g. Savin-Baden, 2000). PBL studies have also indicated how group work builds social understandings and stimulates collaborative learning (Visschers-Pleijers *et al.*, 2004). In this respect, it can be maintained that PBL creates the social capital for the 'private good' as opposed to the 'public good' (Putman, 2000, p. 20). Whereas private forms of social capital are inward looking and reinforce group identity, others are outward looking and encompass people across society – bridging capital. Arguably, PBL groups have the potential to create both, working in the first instance for the good of the group and in preparing students for wider networking in health and social care teams.

There could be challenges where programmes are delivered in a modular format and where students come together from different intellectual fields. In addition, there appears to be no direct evidence as yet that the social capital generated through PBL programmes is sustainable over time, or contributes directly to the public good; although retrospective studies have indicated (e.g. Reeves *et al.*, 2004; see also Chapter 7) that PBL group work, at least for occupational therapy graduates, is influential in developing clinical reasoning skills, team working skills and the confidence of 'neophyte practitioners' (Reeves *et al.*, 2004, p. 326).

PBL and the development of human capital

The creation of human capital can be evidenced through the skills that individuals acquire from the process of higher education. Whilst for example, higher order transferable skills of critical enquiry, reasoned argument and self reflection are not unique to PBL, they are inherent within PBL as a learning process. PBL as a learning method is underpinned by the need for students to engage in self-direction, to demonstrate autonomous learning practices that are designed to reflect the PBL bias towards process rather than content. It is through this ontogenesis of process skills that PBL students are able to cope with change and accrue the human capital beneficial to lifelong learning as well as their professional development. Moreover, there is considerable research in health settings to suggest (e.g. Blumberg & Michael, 1992; Norman & Schmidt, 1992; Sadlo, 1997) that PBL prepares students effectively for lifelong learning.

Conclusion

This chapter has considered how social and human capital are generated through the process of PBL. With reference to the work of Bourdieu, Coleman, Putman and others, we have shown how PBL group work through the promotion of trust, cooperative learning and reciprocity can build the foundations of social capital. It has been argued further that the process skills acquired through the educational approach of PBL offer the human capital necessary to adapt to changing economic and social order. Evidence from health-care literature has been cited to demonstrate the efficacy of PBL in relation to the development of capital. Further research is necessary to illuminate both the development of capital within PBL and also its 'sustainability' over time.

References

Beck, U. (1999) *What Is Globalization*. Polity Press, Cambridge.

Beck, U. (2001) Living your own life in a runaway world: individualism, globalisation and politics. In: *On the Edge: Living with Global Capitalism* (eds W. Hutton & A. Giddens), pp. 164–174. Vintage Books, London.

Becker, G. (1993) *Human Capital: A Theoretical and Empirical Analysis with Special Reference to Education*, 3rd edn. University of Chicago Press, Chicago.

Blumberg, P. & Michael, J.A. (1992) Development of self-directed learning behaviours in a partially, teacher directed problem-based learning curriculum. *Teaching and Learning Medicine.* **1**, 3–8.

Bourdieu, P. (1986) The forms of capital. In: (1997) *Education, Culture, Economy, Society* (eds A.H. Halsey, H. Lauder, P. Brown & A. Stuart Wells), pp. 46–58. Open University Press, Oxford.

Bourdieu, P. (1990) *In Other Words: Essays towards a Reflexive Sociology*. Translated by Matthew Adamson Stanford University Press, Stanford.

Brown, P. (1997) Cultural capital and social exclusion: some observations on recent trends in education, employment, and the labour market. In: *Education, Culture, Economy, Society*. (eds A.H. Halsey, H. Lauder, P. Brown & A. Stuart Wells), pp. 736–749. Open University Press, Oxford.

Coleman, J. (1988) Social capital in the creation of human capital. *American Journal of Sociology.* **94** (Supplement), 95–120.

Coleman, J. (1994) *Foundations of Social Theory*. Harvard University Press, Cambridge, MA.

Dearing, R. (1997) *Summary Report of the UK Committee of Inquiry into Higher Education: Higher Education in the Learning Society*. HMSO, London.

Department of Trade and Industry (1998) *Our Competitive Future: Building the Knowledge Driven Economy*. HMSO, London.

Field, J. (2000) *Lifelong Learning and the New Educational Order*. Trentham Books, London.

Field, J. (2005) *Social Capital and Lifelong Learning*. Routledge, London.

Field, J., Schuller, T. & Baron, S. (2000) Social capital and human capital revisited. In: *Social Capital: Critical Perspectives* (eds S. Baron, J. Field & T. Schuller), pp. 243–264. Oxford University Press, Oxford.

Fine, B. & Green, F. (2000) Economics, social capital, and the colonisation of the social sciences. In: *Social Capital: Critical Perspectives*. (eds S. Baron, J. Field & T. Schuller), pp. 78–94. Oxford University Press, Oxford.

Fukuyama, F. (1999) *The Great Disruption. Human Nature and the Reconstitution of Social Order*. Profile Books Ltd, London.

Giddens, A. (1998) *Consequences of Modernity*. Polity Press, Cambridge.

Grew, R. (2001) Finding social capital: the French revolution in Italy. In: *Patterns of Social Capital Stability and Change in Historical Perspective* (ed. R. Rotberg), pp. 69–95. Cambridge University Press, Cambridge.

Hargreaves, A. (2003) *Teaching in the Knowledge Society: Education in the Age of Insecurity*. Polity Press, Cambridge.

Held, D. & McGrew, A. (2000) The great globalization debate: an introduction. In: *The Global Transformations Reader: An Introduction to the Globalization Debate* (eds D. Held & A. McGrew), pp. 1–45. Polity Press, Cambridge.

Henkel, M. (2000) *Academic Identities and Policy Change in Higher Education*. Jessica Kingsley, London.

Margetson, D. (1994) Current educational reform and the significance of problem-based learning. *Studies in Higher Education*. **19** (1), 5–19.

Norman, G.R. & Schmidt, H.G. (1992) The psychological basis of PBL: a review of the evidence. *Academic Medicine*. **67** (9), 557–565.

Portes, A. (1998) Social capital: its origins and applications in modern sociology. *Annual Review of Sociology*. **24** (1), 1–24.

Pruett, J. & Schwellenbach, N. (2004) *The Rise of Network Universities: Higher Education in the Knowledge Economy*. Paper Presented at the Education, Participation and Globalisation Conference, Prague, 20th–22nd May 2004. Available at: http.72.14.203.104/search/q=cache:MjlrkNC6DwwJ:www.utwatch.org/archives. Accessed on 16th March 2006.

Putman, R. (2000) *Bowling Alone: The Collapse and Revival of American Community*. Simon and Schuster, New York.

Reeves, S. *et al.* (2004) Understanding the effects of problem-based learning on practice: findings from a survey of newly qualified therapists. *British Journal of Occupational Therapy*. **67** (7), 323–327.

Sadlo, G. (1997) Problem-based learning enhances the educational experiences of occupational therapy students. *Education for Health*. **10** (1), 101–114.

Savin-Baden, M. (2000) *Problem-Based Learning in Higher Education: Untold Stories*. Society for Research into Higher Education and the Open University Press, Maidenhead.

Savin-Baden, M. (2003) *Facilitating Problem-Based Learning: Illuminating Perspectives*. Society for Research into Higher Education and the Open University Press, Maidenhead.

Visschers-Pleijers, A.J.S.F. *et al.* (2004) Exploration of a method to analyse group interactions in problem-based learning. *Medical Teacher*. **26** (5), 471–478.

12: An evolving vision for learning in health-care education

Andrew Machon and Gwilym Wyn Roberts

Introduction

This chapter will look at a new and emerging perspective to problem-based learning (PBL), one that is inclusive of both the concepts of appreciative and paradoxical inquiry. Given that the purpose of health-care education is to produce confident, competent and safe practitioners and learners, throughout the chapter we refer to both tutor–student and practitioner–client relationships. The importance of applying transferable skills from education into health- and social-care practice is highlighted, and it seems reasonable therefore that the proposed perspective is potentially and equally valid for both health-care students and qualified practitioners.

Working through PBL develops a strong 'analytical eye' in the student and qualified health practitioner. This is an incisive eye that sees problems and helps to define the solutions. Through PBL, the practitioner takes a detached and objective viewpoint that looks for what is 'broken' and with the help of resources, such as a guiding tutor and a team of students, the research literature and memory, determines the best 'fix' to problem scenarios. In this chapter, we present both the strengths and limitations of PBL. What emerges is how the limitations inherent in PBL create an opportunity for the natural evolution of a complementary learning approach – Appreciative Inquiry (AI). AI is an approach to thinking and learning that works from the propositions of affirmative action and visions of the possible rather than problem solving – finding what is wrong and looking for difficulties (Hammond & Royal, 1998). Therefore, the strengths of AI naturally balance the limitations of PBL.

In contrast to PBL, with its focus on the negative challenge of the problem, AI places its emphasis on the existence of a *positive core*.

From this perspective, development and learning is less determined by problem solving and more a natural consequence of identifying success and what is working well. This approach implies that any problem needs to be considered in the context of what is working well for the client or the case scenario. This may significantly help an understanding of the impact of the problem and its resolution. Whereas PBL places emphasis objectively on finding the problem, AI focuses subjectively on the value and importance of relationship to learning and growth. PBL employs the *analytical eye*, whereas AI necessitates the opening of what we name the *appreciative eye*. If the tutor or practitioner can employ both viewpoints, then vision, practice and learning can be significantly expanded. To evolve how we learn necessitates that the tutor or practitioner cultivates a more integrated and creative vision that accommodates both the analytical and appreciative eyes. This invites both tutors and practitioners alike to work with the dynamic paradox of having both viewpoints in order to realise a multidimensional vision that integrates both these approaches. Even though PBL and AI can be seen as two opposing and starkly contrasting learning approaches, we affirm that one in fact complements the other. They are seen less as two opposing approaches to learning and more as 'two sides' of the same 'coin' of learning. In embracing this, the tutor, student group and practitioner can allow a more creative and relational approach to learning and teaching. This we name as 'Paradoxical Inquiry' (PI).

The value in PI is that it offers and reminds the PBL facilitator or practitioner of the importance of a more unlimited vision and fosters their capacity to work both rationally and relationally. Such an approach and vision integrates an incisive and decisive practical approach together with a more creative, inspirational and relational practice. The PI learning approach is introduced and outlined. The implications of PI are considered in the additional skills that it offers the tutor and the student practitioner. We explore how this integrative context and approach to learning will both serve and motivate higher level practice. Also, how these new and emerging skills together ensure a deepening awareness of the importance of the tutor–student and practitioner–client relationship. In addition, we consider how this may positively inform and influence the culture of health-care education and practice.

The analytical eye – a one-dimensional (1D) vision of learning

PBL invites the student and health-care practitioner to show personal initiative by defining their specific learning needs. Using their own experience together with a team as a resource, these practitioners define the information needed to inform and essentially solve the problem in hand. It is clear that this opportunity for self-directed learning within

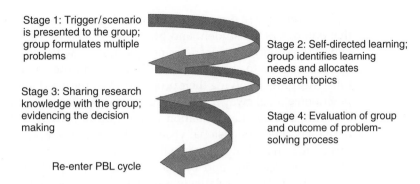

Stage 1: Trigger/scenario is presented to the group; group formulates multiple problems

Stage 2: Self-directed learning; group identifies learning needs and allocates research topics

Stage 3: Sharing research knowledge with the group; evidencing the decision making

Stage 4: Evaluation of group and outcome of problem-solving process

Re-enter PBL cycle

The focus remains on solving the problem

Figure 12.1   A traditional PBL approach.

the context of solving a problem marks a distinctive development and progress from the more traditional subject-based didactic teaching method. What PBL specifically cultivates is an objective, critical and 'analytical eye' that sees largely problems and their solution. An illustration of a traditional PBL approach to problem solving is illustrated in Figure 12.1. The problem, be it a scenario in teaching or one faced by the client in practice, is viewed objectively from a detached analytical and rational viewpoint. The focus is upon the factual and practical that is commonly assessed in terms of measurable outcomes. A critical appraisal and diagnosis is made of the situation and commonly, the practitioner defines and critically judges what is needed to solve the problem faced by the client. The goal is an intervention where the practitioner solves the problem by helping the client in someway to adapt. What is commonly missed or devalued is the actual role of the client in problem assessment and its solution which is as follows:

▪ What is currently working well for the client?
▪ How does the client assess this particular problem relative to what appears to be working well?
▪ How is the problem weighed against others?
▪ Does this problem hide a further deeper challenge that they face?
▪ How might they actively engage in the problem's resolution in a true client-centred manner?

These questions can at times be devalued and overlooked in the PBL approach, if the power to solve is seen to reside predominantly with the practitioner. It is important to consider the nature of the problem-solving approach that PBL employs. The analytical eye is fast incisive and decisive. It quickly and critically evaluates and then defines the solution commonly from memory.

PBL is therefore a directive approach to learning and problem solving that empowers the student and practitioner to solve the client's problems. An important reflection and question is whether empowering the practitioner to solve, in turn, disempowers the client from more fully engaging in solving their problem? Does the good intention of the practitioner steal away a vital source of learning from the client?

A further potential limitation of the PBL approach is the narrow, partial and one-dimensional vision of the analytical eye. As discussed earlier, the analytical eye, critically and objectively observes the world of teaching, learning and practice as one of the problems that need to be solved. This is relatively a narrow and superficial vision. There is evidence that the focus of our intervention prior to taking action influences the outcome that we find. Hawkins (2006) reminds the tutor and the practitioner that one's range of choice is ordinarily limited only by one's vision. In line with this view, Hammond (1998) notes, that if we look only for problems, then that is what we will find. This infers that employing only the 'analytical eye' that looks for problems merely results in finding more problems to be solved. One potential danger with this approach is the preoccupation of the tutor or practitioner with problem solving. In the PBL approach, the tutor or practitioner can overlook the importance of what are working well and the fuller engagement of the client in resolving their own problems. Cloke and Goldsmith (2003, p. 179) suggest that we consider a most pertinent question: 'are we able to resist the narcotic of problem solving?' For as Hammond (1998, p. 9) notes, 'we are obsessed with learning from our mistakes'. In essence, we need to consider to what degree are we capable of letting things happen or do we seek either knowing or unknowingly, to control the process? Furthermore, might the habitual solving of problems inhibit a deeper possible learning of the client that is essential to their growth and development? If we can resist the temptation to urgently solve the problem, might we then engage the client more fully in the process? A potential danger expressed by Cloke and Goldsmith (2003, p. 180) is that:

> in thinking that we know the one correct answer and in deciding to enlarge our ego's, we do so at the cost of reduced skills in the person who has to live with the result.

It is important here that we do not throw out 'the baby with the bath water'. We do not deny the great value of the technical expertise and very practical need and role of the health-care worker or the value of problem solving. However, might our detached objectivity devalue the importance of the subjective experience of the practitioner–client relationship? The objective, determinate and rational approach fostered by PBL can overlook the importance of seeing the client beyond the immediate problem that they present. It may be more common in practice than we realise that the presented problem is not the major problem of importance to the client. The question this raises is what is the ideal balance between the application of technical expert skills and the ability and competency of the practitioner to engage and relate more deeply and to assess and appreciate the needs of the client? How important is our ability to relate and the quality of the relationships that we build with the client? To what degree do we actually engage the client in the problem-solving process; are we able to see the client separate from the problem that we believe needs to be addressed? One of the potential limitations of PBL is that the rational approach it fosters tends to keep the student in their 'heads' and unaware of matters of 'heart'.

The 'heart' is more the realm of a more appreciative and relational approach. The critical, objective and determinate nature of the 'analytical eye' creates a dispassionate view where the client is known objectively from the outside looking in and it remains a mystery who they are and what they may need as seen from the inside looking out. This can foster a negative attitude and culture of seeing the client as a problem needing to be solved. Edmonstone (2006) notes how this focus on what is not working may reduce morale through creating the sense of a problem-filled environment. The key limitation of PBL is not therefore its analytical and rational process of problem solving that certainly has an important place and practical value. It is more the limited context or vision of the analytical eye that may blindly overlook the need to relate and more fully engage with the client in order to further their ownership of the problem and learning. What value does the health-care practitioner place on relating to their client and understanding their needs from the inside out? Is an objective and 'analytical eye' alone adequate and appropriate to the learning, practice and culture of health care that the tutor and practitioner ultimately creates?

The 'appreciative eye' – a two-dimensional (2D) vision of learning

It is not in our view a chance occurrence that AI is emerging as a contrasting, valuable and insightful approach to learning. It is the limitations of PBL if owned, that informs the emergent strengths and potential learning through AI. These two approaches are naturally complementary, even though most commonly, they are viewed as two independent and starkly contrasting approaches to learning. AI invites a different context and vision to that of PBL. In contrast to developing the 'analytical eye', AI instead cultivates the 'appreciative eye'. AI invites the teacher or practitioner to become more aware of and to engage with and discover – a 'positive core'. This is a source of the student and client's potential learning and growth. This core is a source of motivation and aspiration and as such indicates the direction of their future success and fulfilment. AI assumes that such a positive learning experience comes from identifying, emphasising and seeking to replicate what is working well (Edmonstone, 2006). Whereas PBL sees the nature of one's problem as finding that which is 'broken' and fixing it, AI sees what is already working well and places energy and emphasis there. This invites the health-care practitioner to enter into relationship with the client in order to share in the discovery of the client's source of yet unrealised potential and growth. The invitation through AI is to relate with the client in order to appreciate their success, passions and future aspirations. This deeper, more relational and subjective awareness becomes the fertile context in which to consider the apparent 'problem' that they face and how it might best be resolved.

Note that in contrast to PBL and its active problem-solving role for the student and qualified practitioner, AI invites the practitioner to be a more non-directive, relational facilitator. Whereas PBL is problem orientated, placing power and emphasis on the practitioner to solve, the AI approach is a much more reflective question-orientated approach. This engages and affirms the power of the student and client to learn and resolve for themselves. In employing AI, the power is placed back with the student and client to define their learning needs by owning and learning from their problems in the context of their wider aspirations. PBL cultivates a culture where the tutor and/or practitioner are empowered to teach or solve, respectively. In contrast, AI acknowledges the clients as the expert of their own learning and the practitioner as a facilitator of this possibility. In the AI approach, the answer to their learning and continued growth ever rests with the student or client. If we take away the chance to problem solve away, we steal a profound opportunity for personal empowerment and learning. Through the appreciative eye, the importance of the problem and the need to solve may often diminish. AI does not ignore the problem but chooses instead to invest energy very largely in what is working well. Jung (1967, p. 15) noted that:

> the greatest and most important problems in life are all in a certain sense insoluble. They must be so because they express the necessary polarity inherent in every self-regulating system. They can never be solved . . . only outgrown.

This insight points towards a deeper paradox inherent within our concept of the problem. What Jung implies is rather than solving our problems, might they if viewed as a source of personal learning, foster growth? The urgency to solve may steal the chance to learn through and grow from exploring the problem.

Paradoxical inquiry (PI) – an evolving (3D) vision of learning

As we explore deeper into the nature of ourselves and how we learn, we are met with paradox. A quote from the beginning of Foucault's pendulum (Eco, 1990, p. 95) expressed this realisation well:

> I have come to believe that the whole world is an enigma, a harmless enigma that is made terrible by our own mad attempt to interpret it as though it had an underlying truth.

So how might an understanding of paradox inform and evolve our approach to learning? A paradox is the natural existence of contradictory realities. This invites the reader to consider if our problems are more complex and multidimensional than our rational thinking would have us perceive. In our urgent need to solve our problems, do we oversimplify and steal the chance away to contemplate and learn more deeply from the dilemma they present? Might the appreciation of these deeper dilemmas guide us towards new resolutions or a more elegant and balanced solution? The analytical eye is ever intent on critically judging what is 'right or wrong' and so simplifying and solving problems. Paradox with its innate contradiction suggests that there may always be more than one possibility.

Paradox therefore invites the rational mind and how we think and the 'analytical eye' and how we see, to resist the temptation to solve, in order to appreciate and embrace contradiction and dilemma as a natural aspect of life, reality and how we learn. It is not possible to rational solve a paradox; it can only be embraced. If we can learn however, to expand our vision to see paradox, might we also learn how to extend our thinking beyond the rational? Paradox if we own it, may offer a secret alchemy that can transform our urgency to solve into a deeper, more imaginative and creative curiosity (Machon, 2005). If the rational mind can be taught patience by paradox, then we may be given the chance to more deeply reflect upon our apparent problems and their dilemmas. This would provide the opportunity to more deeply 'mine' our problems purely for their learning. If we can learn to see our problems as more than something to be swiftly solved, then they can guide us to consider our vital questions. When the urgency to solve is taken away, we are free to relate more fully with our students and clients and can also remember our motivations – the person we long to be and become. In our ability to reflect and question, we can remember the larger context of our aspirations and those of our clients. Problems become less of an obstacle to be solved and more a guide to our motivations that inspire our growth and learning. If we can learn to resist the need to solve, our problems can guide us to consider the larger context in which they may be resolved. In this way, rather than solving our problems, we can explore their deeper meaning and value to our lives. One might even consider if our problems hold the only key to our vital learning and growth. Paradox reminds that we can learn through our problems, if we can resist the temptation to solve them. As health- and social-care practitioners, we may need to realise and remember the importance of our questions relative to our answers. It is through the question that our client's aspirations can blossom. A quick solution can slam a door on the chance to ask and reflect upon these vital questions. If we do seek to solve quickly and ignore the underlying paradox of the problem, we may in fact exacerbate the real problem rather than alleviate it.

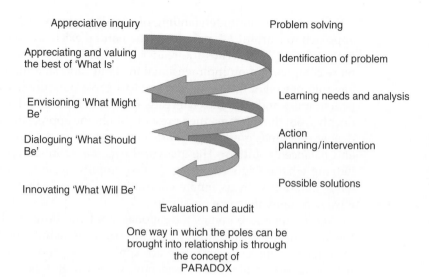

Appreciative inquiry   Problem solving

Appreciating and valuing   Identification of problem
the best of 'What Is'

Envisioning 'What Might   Learning needs and analysis
Be'

Dialoguing 'What Should   Action
Be'   planning/intervention

Innovating 'What Will Be'   Possible solutions

Evaluation and audit

One way in which the poles can be
brought into relationship is through
the concept of
PARADOX

Figure 12.2   Integrating PBL and AI. Adapted from Cooperrider and Srivastava (1987).

What paradox teaches is the importance of expanding and integrating our vision as tutors and practitioners by combining the 'analytical and appreciative eyes' innate to the PBL and AI approaches respectively. What additional value might we find if we could see these approaches not as distinct and separate entities but more as two sides of the same 'coin of learning'? Can we in integrating these approaches (Figure 12.2) make problem solving less of a compulsion and more a choice, empowering the client to learn more deeply and grow by actively engaging with and helping resolve their problems?

The analytical eye is focused on finding the answer. When we employ the analytical eye, the role of the practitioner is more as a tutor or instructor. The inclusion of the 'appreciative eye' shifts the role of the tutor and practitioner from one of an active problem solver to more of a questioning and listening facilitator. Rather than seeking the answer, the opening of the appreciative eye gives the tutor or practitioner the chance to explore the value of the question. In addition, the appreciative eye is a sensing as well as a seeing eye; it is keen to listen as well as observe and so is able to relate with empathy. The vision of the appreciative eye therefore extends awareness beyond self to embrace a deeper appreciation of the other. This learning approach therefore invites the tutor and practitioner to include and maximise the value of learning through the therapist–client or student–tutor relationship. What this integrative approach to learning does is to place centrally and equally the importance of the vital question, the quality of how we relate with our clients, as well as the need (at the appropriate time) to focus, solve and decide. The implication of this approach is that a deeper learning can be gained by consciously working with both the analytical and appreciative eyes. This integration of PBL and AI to bring a third learning approach PI evolves a three-dimensional vision of learning. This further step happens through the opening of what we name as the creative eye. The lens of this creative eye can engage either or both the analytical and appreciative eyes and yet has a dynamic flexibility to listen, question, relate and resolve.

What PI uniquely offers is a dynamic flexibility of response with an ability to balance the capacity of practitioner to both relate and/or solve as is required. This has the potential for a much more flexible, innovative and creative response. The dynamic flexibility of the creative eye is expressed in Figure 12.3. When we integrate these learning approaches into PI, what we gain is a major shift in our approach to learning. Whereas PBL seeks to find and solve the problem, PI reminds and offers the practitioner the chance to expand their awareness of the current problem. The chance to expand awareness in this way allows the practitioner to verify whether this is the key problem faced by the client, how they might engage and learn through the solving of the problem and how the aspirations of the client might reframe this problem. This places an initial emphasis on the AI approach and primarily the engagement of the appreciative eye to more deeply relate to the client. Problem solving becomes decentralised. What PI offers is less of problem-focused approach but much more of a solution-focused approach where the technical skills of the practitioner are married with the personal understanding and expertise of the client. It is from this context that the presenting problem finds its true value and meaning. From this relational positioning, the health-care practitioner can then further engage with the client to explore how they may wish or seek to resolve the problem for themselves. Having established this breadth and scope of information relative to the presenting problem, the practitioner can then engage the analytical eye to how they might

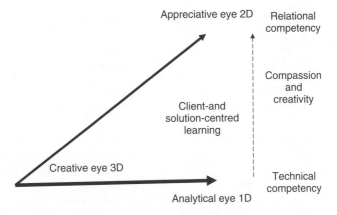

Figure 12.3 Opening the creative eye of paradoxical inquiry.

best help resolve the problem together with the client. The PI approach is diagrammatically presented in Figure 12.3. What happens through the use of PI is that one's vision and awareness of the problem is first expanded through different ways of seeing, sensing and thinking, extending the client and practitioner's capacity for learning, and the finding when required, of more creative and compassionate solution. Throughout, the PI approach ensures that the client and not the practitioner is centrally empowered in the process of finding solutions and learning.

In applying what we may imagine to be a more flexible lens to finding solutions, the client takes responsibility to frame the importance of the apparent problem, to engage and learn and to make meaning for themselves – which may form a new and key aspect of problem resolution and client-centred practice. The approach of PI to learning invites the tutor, student and so eventually the practitioner, to become a relational facilitator and a solution-focused problem solver. This shifting role of the tutor practitioner from instructor to a relational facilitator and technical expert will essentially develop and inform higher level practice. This approach is truly client-centred and yet equally invites the application of the technical expertise of practice. The relational competencies of the student are valued equally to their practical ability. The use of PI will evolve new practitioners who have cultivated both relational and technical competencies and balance both equally, and who will in turn potentially influence the culture of health care. Perceptions of today's health-care system suggest that it is one where the analytical approach may be key. Practitioners may be constrained to operate with the particular presenting problem and are not invited to relate more deeply with the client as a context in which to more fully learn and more creatively and elegantly resolve problems. Might it be a valued intention that part of the role of learning and

Table 12.1 The contrasting viewpoints of the analytical, appreciative and creative eyes.

Viewpoint	Characteristics	Concept of problem
Analytical eye Problem-focused PBL	Objective, critical, judging, detached	Seeks problems and their solution
Appreciative eye Client-centred AI	Subjective, relational	Problem is a prompt to the larger context of what is working well for the client
Creative eye Client- and solution-focused PI	Creative, relational, rational	Problem is key to the clients' potential for learning and growth

teaching is to also mindfully create a culture of health care that places the needs of the client's health and learning as essential and central? PI has the capacity as an approach, to extend the vision of learning and practice, whilst positively influencing a potential culture change within higher education and the health-care system. Such may be the fulfilment of allowing our vision of learning to evolve in health-care teaching and practice (Table 12.1).

How can we foster the use of PI? What support do our tutors and practitioners need?

Key to the evolution of learning is how we can support the use and application of these new learning approaches in the work of both the tutor and practitioner. What we need to do is to be able to have a supervisory support that can work with the evolving eye necessary to maximising learning and growth. Supervisors need to be comfortable in working with the relative and collective value of the analytical, appreciative and creative eye in practice.

As well as technical skills, such supervision needs to employ an expert level of relational and rational intelligence. The role of the practitioner in cultivating learning is shifting from one of instructor and technical expert to one of facilitator and coach. It is important to consider how supervision needs to accommodate and appreciate the shifting role and the importance of the ability to coach and facilitate in order to maximise our own and our clients' learning. This is an important consideration. How different might the fulfilment of our clients and practitioners be if we could implement this approach to learning in health care? It would necessitate that the fulfilment and learning of our clients are valued equally to the more measurable outcomes of our expert technical practice. This evolving vision of learning might both inspire a culture that supports our continued learning and practice.

References

Cloke, K. & Goldsmith, J. (2003) *The Art of Waking People Up: Cultivating Awareness and Authenticity at Work*. Jossey-Bass, San Franscisco.

Cooperrider, D. & Srivastava, R. (1987) Appreciative inquiry in organizational life. In: *Research on Organizational Change and Development*, Vol. 1 (eds T. Woodman & M. Pasmore), pp. 129–169. JA1 Press, S.A.

Eco, U. (1990) *Foucault's Pendulum. Gruppo Editoriale Fabbri Bompiani Sonzogno*. Etas, Milano.

Edmonstone, J. (2006) *Building on the Best: An Introduction to Appreciative Inquiry in Healthcare*. Kingsham Press, London.

Hammond, S.A. (1998) *The Thin Book of Appreciative Inquiry*. Thin Book Publishing Company, Plano, TX.

Hammond, S. & Royal, C. (1998) *Lessons from the Field: Applying Appreciative Inquiry.* Thin Book Publishing, Plano, TX.

Hawkins, D.R. (2006) *Power vs Force: The Hidden Determinants of Human Behaviour.* Hay House UK limited, London.

Jung, C.G. (1967) *Commentary on 'The Secret Golden Flower' in Collected Works,* Vol. 13. Routledge and Kegan Paul, London.

Machon, A. (2005) *Just Beyond the Visible: The Art of Being and Becoming.* Arem Publishing, London.

Part 3

The Learner in Problem-Based Learning

13: The student experience

Liz Galle and Sandra Marshman

Introduction

The authors of this chapter are two former occupational therapy students who undertook a full-time 3-year problem-based learning (PBL) programme. Our intentions for this chapter are to provide a students' perspective: what it felt like being part of the PBL process, what was good about it and what not so good. We explore how PBL contrasted with our previous learning experiences and how we felt the programme prepared us to move forward into practice.

As authors, we have used 'I' when describing our individual experience and reflections and 'we' when our comments are drawn from our combined experiences and shared opinions. This has allowed us to offer our subjective and intersubjective experiences, and we hope this helps you as readers to follow our journey through the PBL process.

The chapter takes Savin-Baden's (2000) *Dimensions of Learner Experience*, which emerged from her empirical study exploring staff and students' experience of PBL, as a framework to structure the account. Using this framework also enables comparisons to be drawn between the findings of the study in which Savin-Baden (2000) describes concepts termed *stances* and the authors' perceptions of the student experience. Furthermore, by integrating the research findings into this chapter, the intention is to encourage a deeper level of analysis of what is a personal account of two students' experiences of PBL.

Firstly, the framework *Dimensions of Learner Experience* will be described and the personal account will then be structured through the three concepts emerging from the research: personal stance, pedagogical stance and interactional stance.

Dimensions of learner experience

The research by Maggi Savin-Baden was undertaken with four distinct professional groups in four British universities from 1991 to 1995.

Each department had implemented PBL in some way. Three concepts were felt to capture the complexity and paradox across the sites; these emerged from people's experiences of PBL and they are defined as follows:

▪ Personal stance: the way in which staff and students see themselves in relation to the learning context and give their own distinctive meaning to their experience of that context.
▪ Pedagogical stance: the ways in which people see themselves as learners in particular educational environments.
▪ Interactional stance: the ways in which learners work and learn in groups and construct meaning in relation to one another (Savin-Baden, 2000, p. 55).

These concepts form the framework termed *Dimensions of Learner Experience*; they are interrelated and together capture the multifaceted nature of the learner experience (Savin-Baden, 2000).

Personal stance

A contrast to previous learning experiences

Within PBL, personal stance refers to the interplay between what students bring to and take from their learning experiences, the way they speak about themselves, and view their profession, their peers, the facilitator and the institution (Savin-Baden, 2000).

Despite the written and verbal information and the 'mock' PBL group experiences at the entrance interview, I have since reflected that on entry to the course, I did not have more than a basic overview of what PBL involved and how it differentiated from traditional programmes of education. Undertaking professional training again was exciting and I felt privileged to have the opportunity to engage with this new discipline; however, becoming a student again filled me with dread. My previous experience of student nurse training 21 years ago, was of sitting in a classroom, in rows, in uniform, waiting to be taught all I needed to know. The contrast with a PBL environment could not have been more striking. We were in a small group, about eight of us looking at a case study of a young homeless man. It quickly became apparent that there were no immediate 'right' answers to be uncovered with which to 'solve' his problems; we were to go away and explore the issues the case study generated and feed these back to the group.

The experience of transition, from a traditional learning environment to a PBL group, left me feeling unsure of what was expected. Within the personal stance Savin-Baden (2000) suggests that *fragmentation* occurs, as within PBL, students are responsible for deciding what constitutes relevant learning, they are encouraged to decide what counts as knowledge, and experience the role of tutor differently. These challenges to values and beliefs can lead to a sense of fragmentation. This was a difficult time of wanting more guidance and having the expectation that tutors would confirm whether knowledge fed back was that knowledge which 'they' the tutors intended to be found. When this confirmation did not happen, or was confused by several alternative approaches to solve the 'problem', it increased the sense of uncertainty.

Disjunction, a concept taken from Jarvis, 1987 and Weil, 1989, is described by Savin-Baden (2000) as referring to 'a sense of fragmentation of part of, or all of the self, characterised by frustration and confusion, and a loss of sense of self; and often resulting in anger, frustration, and a desire for "right" answers' (Savin-Baden, 2000, p. 87). Many students were angry and it was difficult not to be influenced by this pervading feeling. However, previous experience of working within health care taught me that within the complexities of practice, finding 'right answers' was not straightforward or even possible. As Rolfe (1998) suggests, even in the hard sciences, we can never be *absolutely* certain about what is known, nevertheless, in science we do have reasonable grounds to suppose that the future will resemble the past, unlike in health and social care, where the behaviour of individual people is far from predictable. I was aware of and had experienced knowledge evolving as research informed theory and practice. Being able, in these early months, to embrace a certain level of uncertainty as we encountered 'real life' scenarios in the classroom, greatly reduced feelings of frustration and disjunction at this time.

Valuing prior experience

My fears about becoming a student again quickly diminished; this was largely due to the group facilitators actively enquiring about group members' prior experience and being encouraged to share knowledge within the group. It has been suggested that activation of prior knowledge facilitates the subsequent processing of new information and often occurs within PBL groups (Norman & Schmidt, 1992). This process of sharing something of myself with others helped me to integrate who I was, with who I was becoming. My concern about starting afresh diminished and was replaced by the feeling that I was able to build upon existing knowledge, it was still of value, and the sharing and discussion provided an important means of connection between my existing self and my new developing self. Valuing and acknowledging prior experience is considered a key component of PBL (Barrows & Tamblyn, 1980). We feel this is an important strength of PBL, and believe we would not have felt the same level of motivation and self-affirmation had we been taught by a lecture-based method that did not require exploration of prior learning and interchange of ideas. We felt personally involved with the learning process right from the beginning.

A new way of being

Maintaining this connection between my former and developing self, helped me to feel more secure during this period of rapid change and personal growth. Savin-Baden (2000) suggests that students develop a heightened understanding of their own reality because of the relationship between previous and new experiences. I had the thought during these early months, that here was an opportunity to change and develop into who I wanted to become. As I engaged with new ideas, I felt I could keep aspects that were of value and were important links to my new self, but I could also discard those parts that I disliked and had no further use for. It felt as if I was experimenting with new ways of being. Though this presented an opportunity for change, I was conscious of becoming more self-aware and as I contributed within the group and appraised others' responses towards me, this caused uncomfortable feelings as it challenged my sense of self. Savin-Baden (2000) writes of transitions – shifts in learner experience that are often sites of struggle but carries with them the idea of movement and the necessity of taking up a new position in a different place. As the course progressed, how I placed myself in relation to new concepts and as my feelings towards previously held values and beliefs became more stable, I was able to identify more clearly with this new way of being.

Habermas (1989) developed the approach that it is through the action of communicating that society actually operates and evolves – a process encompassed and structured by the actors' life-worlds. These communicative actions he suggests, are the ways that people develop, confirm and renew their memberships in social groups, and develop their own identities. Finlay (1998) describes a person's life-world as pertaining to individual meanings and habits as we exist in a world filled with complex meanings, which form the backdrop of our everyday actions and interactions. It is suggested that PBL challenges students to confront the relationship between the previous experiences of their life-world and their new experiences, which can lead to new understandings; thus, students might speak of inner resonance between their life-world and what they were learning (Savin-Baden, 2000).

Pedagogical stance

Students' pedagogical stance is described as the way in which students see themselves as learners, developed from a combination of prior learning experiences, their assumed notions of learning and teaching and the type of higher education they receive (Savin-Baden, 2000).

Adjusting to problem-based learning

Being part of the experience of PBL, though a marked contrast to previous learning, had the effect of affirming values and beliefs. We felt able to take responsibility for our own learning, and the discovery that this was an expectation that was met with a sense of relief. This was going to be different. In addition, we felt there was a belief in our abilities as students to discover for ourselves, which increased our confidence and had the effect of motivating us further.

This was not the case for all students; there was the feeling expressed by some that we had been abandoned, this was DIY learning and resentment developed. Comments voiced in the early months were that we were not being taught; it was being left to us to do the work and find things out. Savin-Baden (2000) suggests that students within 'reproductive pedagogy' may revert to methods of learning that they have always used: They expect learning to be safe and predictable, requiring neither personal initiative nor critical thought; teachers are seen to be the suppliers of all legitimate knowledge. Learning about the theory of PBL early on in the course helped to relieve some of the uncertainty and unexpectedness that was encountered. It has been suggested that PBL is the most basic human learning process that allowed primitive man to survive in his environment; facts related to us by others rarely seem to have the tenacity of the information we have gained from our own daily confrontation with problems (Barrows & Tamblyn, 1980). By working on problems as simulations of 'real life' situations, it seemed from the outset that we were being encouraged to think as a practitioner would and this generated a feeling of anticipation of becoming that person. A key feature of PBL therefore, is the assumption that learning takes place most effectively when students are actively involved and learn in the context in which knowledge is to be used. Comments from participants in a study exploring student perceptions about self-directed learning within a PBL programme would seem to reflect this: 'Feeling responsible and independent at the same time motivated me to increase my knowledge' and 'one acquires merit and self-esteem when one looks and learns by oneself' (Ryan, 1993, p. 61).

Though we enjoyed the freedom of taking control over aspects of our learning, for some, a lack of direction could be daunting. Cornwall (1998, p. 245) suggested of students transferring to self-directed learning programmes that too much independence can lead to sinking rather than learning to swim, and he states: 'independence, like freedom, needs a framework to nurture and support it.' It would seem therefore, that there is a delicate balance to be achieved between promoting self-direction while providing a supportive environment where students feel secure enough to learn.

Placement experience

From a pedagogical point of view, the experience of placements for us created a disabling disjunction; we felt we were following an apprenticeship model of learning and there was the expectation that we would arrive with a defined body of knowledge ready to be applied to the setting. The fact that we were able to seek out information appeared to be less valued. The research undertaken by Savin-Baden (2000) highlighted that many nurse practitioners were socialising students into the apprenticeship model of learning where student nurses were not expected to think and reflect, but to do as they were told. It seemed that within the apprenticeship model, there were power differences that were less obvious within the PBL environment experienced at university; this felt disabling and inhibited self-direction and autonomy in learning. Weil (1989) describes disjuncture as the feeling of being at odds with oneself; this may be in relation to dealing with multiple and conflicting roles and the ways in which social and power differences were experienced and managed.

We felt PBL encouraged us to adopt a reflective pedagogy (Savin-Baden, 2000) where learning involved not only critically evaluating knowledge but also the values implicit within that knowledge. Savin-Baden (2000, p. 63) suggests students in this domain perceive that there are valid perspectives other than their own and accept that 'all kinds of knowing can help them to "know" the world better.' We remember with unease sometimes doubting the value of the contribution made by school leavers on the course and having to reappraise this opinion and learn from the experiences they shared. We felt we were open to others' perspectives on placement and though learning took place apprenticeship-style, we learnt much professional craft knowledge. However, we felt we adopted the role of student that was being expected of us, a 'strategic pedagogy' described in Savin-Baden's study as that which happens when students choose to embrace the perceptions of staff expectations in order to pass the placement.

Interactional stance

Interactional stance is described by Savin-Baden (2000) as the way in which a learner interacts with others in a learning situation, the relationships between students within groups and facilitator–student relationships.

Developing a professional identity

Undertaking professional education required engaging with a new ideology and creating a new identity within this culture. It is suggested that problem-based approaches to professional education provide initial enculturation by providing the earliest communities of practice (Walker, 2001). PBL facilitated this process of enculturation in a way my previous experience of didactic teaching methods did not. Being taught about the values and beliefs inherent in a profession was very different to actively discovering and beginning the process of taking ownership of them. This feeling of owning the discovered knowledge, and possibly having to defend it, was then reinforced when feeding back to the group for debate and discussion. I feel the active participation facilitated my personal development, considered a key part of becoming and developing as a professional (Titchen & Higgs, 2001). I was beginning to know myself in a different way as this new identity developed.

Styles of facilitation

Active participation in the PBL groups was only possible because of the facilitative style of the tutor. They supported and encouraged the learner to question, delve deeper and justify their learning. I can remember thinking that as facilitators were developing person-centred and empowering relationships with us as students, so I would want to develop similar relationships with clients in practice. It seemed appropriate therefore that education should mirror these fundamental values (Carnall, 1998). I experienced the 'liberating' effect of feeling that my judgements were as valid as those of the facilitators (Brookfield, 1986), and I appreciated the mutual respect that developed when facilitators enabled this to happen by sharing their 'power' with us in this way.

However difficulties were encountered, we remember feeling frustrated with ambiguous answers from tutors when it was felt we needed confirmation. Sometimes tutors did not seem in tune with how we struggled with the process. Also, there were times when it seemed appropriate to consider them a resource but this was not always an option available to us. Also, tutors' styles of facilitation differed. Some were more directive, others less so. It is suggested, within PBL groups that, facilitation encompasses guiding 'learners through their own discovery without teaching in the traditional sense' (Biley & Smith, 1999, p. 1205; Clouston, 2005). To expand the definition, facilitation has been described as:

> A goal-orientated dynamic process in which participants work together in an atmosphere of genuine mutual respect, in order to learn through critical reflection.
>
> (Burrows, 1997, p. 401)

However, there could be feelings of frustration at times if tutors seemed to be holding back information just for the sake of 'not telling' (Clouston, 2005). Because I had been a nurse before, I had a distinct advantage and I can remember becoming suddenly very useful as a resource. However, I could appreciate my popularity at the beginning of the course was because I was giving out as much information as I knew, which was seen to be the exact opposite to the stance taken by the facilitators, who were seen as 'withholding', and were consequently viewed less favourably. Data from interviews (Ryan, 1997; Clouston, 2005) suggested that students were at times critical of the role that the tutors had adopted – that is, to consistently reflect knowledge questions back to the student for exploration as self-directed learning; however, it can be argued that this is a necessary strategy when the overt aim is to have students assume responsibility for learning. Ryan suggests however, that there is the question of balance between the expectation that students will find the information for themselves, and the tutor acting as resource person; it can, he suggests, be difficult to get the balance 'right'. Furthermore, opinions vary as to the desirable level of intervention by the PBL facilitator, ranging from active involvement in, to silent observer of the process; evidence suggests there is a very fine balance between tactical intervention and a heavy-handed overly didactic approach (Haith-Cooper, 2000; Clouston, 2005). Learning seemed to be most successful when facilitators were felt to be genuine and honest with us, showed interest in our discussions and shared their opinions. Taylor and Burgess (1997) writing with reference to students entering higher education through non-traditional routes, suggest that there are important integrating factors that mitigate against feelings of disjuncture, key among these being positive valuing of students both by facilitators and peers within learning groups.

The group experience

Savin-Baden (2000) suggests within her study that within the interactional stance, there is an ethic of individualism, that students despite acknowledging that they need to work as a group to develop skills in teamwork, opt for individualism to improve their chances of better grades. Producing work collectively could feel frustrating, particularly if not all group members were as committed to the task. However, we did gain much personal insight from the roles we adopted within these groups. Savin-Baden (1997) suggests that students learn through reflection on the group process as much as through the content under discussion. Furthermore, it is suggested that through the experience of being heard within a group, students learn to value their own knowledge and experience; this learning for some holding more meaning than learning that was rewarded through assessment (Savin-Baden, 2000).

We valued the mutual support that developed, while simultaneously developing some mediation skills. This was reflected in Savin-Baden's study where a student talked of learning about democracy, loyalty and effective teamwork, a process encapsulated by engaging with the life-worlds of others and through reflection, relating other life-worlds to his own. We were conscious of multiple processes at play within the group; we were aware of continually evaluating our performance, whilst also engaging with new concepts. This greater self-awareness has been beneficial in working life where collaboration on tasks has often been required. Within the course, team projects were not assessed, and this went a long way to reducing conflicts. Though we preferred presenting work as part of a group, we enjoyed the opportunities to produce assignments, which were individually assessed. It was often a pleasant relief to be working on something without needing to check it out with the group.

Moving into practice

Savin-Baden (2000) suggests that PBL intends to equip students to become questioning and critical practitioners – practitioners who would not only evaluate themselves and their peers effectively, but would also be able to analyse the shortcomings of policy and practice.

In addition, students work with problem scenarios based on real clinical situations in preparation for the realities and complexities of the workplace and undertake learning in groups which mirrors the situation in the real world where practitioners work as members of a team (Creedy & Alavi, 1997). The emphasis placed on self-direction within the PBL philosophy encourages skills conducive to lifelong learning (Glen, 1995). As practitioners working within the constantly changing nature of health care, we believe PBL helped us to approach change openly and flexibly, and appreciate that there are many ways of knowing within health care. We feel group work within PBL prepared us well for multidisciplinary team working as practitioners explore the complex issues presented. In addition, we feel we have developed the ability to assertively seek out knowledge and critically appraise its worth.

This confidence has taken some time to develop, however, there was the feeling on initially entering the profession, that we lacked a knowledge base. It is suggested that the knowledge that clinicians bring to the clinical encounter takes three forms: propositional, theoretical or scientific knowledge; professional craft knowledge or knowing how to do something and personal knowledge about oneself as a person and in relation with others (Higgs & Titchen, 1995). On qualifying, to possess professional craft knowledge seemed of most relevance 'to know how' to do something and there was the feeling that others in practice who had received traditional training had a sound knowledge base that had been provided for them so they knew the 'right' way to act. It was a time when uncertainties about PBL returned and we wondered if we had learnt enough to be competent. It is suggested however, that within PBL, there may be several models in operation; within a model of PBL that emphasises the development of skills and competencies to manage complexities, this can downgrade the understanding of what it means to be a professional and offers the student the notion that the professional is someone who has a tool kit of skills to apply to any situation (Savin-Baden, 2000). It is suggested however, that skills and know-how are not to be thrown out if this model is to be adopted, but concepts need to be rooted in the notion of 'skills *with* cognitive content and professional judgement' (Savin-Baden, 2000, p. 129). Though entering practice was a stressful time, we believe PBL equipped us with a strong sense of personal responsibility, good team working skills and confidence in a climate of change.

Conclusion

This chapter has used Savin-Baden's (2000) *Dimensions of Learner Experience* to provide a framework to explore what it was like to be a student on a PBL course. Within the personal stance, I experienced the marked difference between my prior experience of traditional training where learning involved being the recipient of knowledge and PBL which required active participation in seeking and defining what counted as knowledge. This initially caused a barrier to learning, a feeling of disjunction; however the realisation that prior knowledge was still important in this process created a shift towards integration, and feelings of curiosity for this way of learning developed. Within the pedagogical stance, it can be said that PBL encourages flexibility and the valuing of other perspectives so that students are more ready to adapt to changing work environments. The interactional stance captures the way learners interact with each other and the facilitator. Learning seemed to be most successful when facilitators were felt to be genuine and honest with us, not withholding information or being too directive, but sharing our enthusiasm for discovery. We found we were developing a new way of being as we discovered a greater self-knowledge through the group process and through active participation in engaging with the values and beliefs of the profession. Of most importance, we felt our experience of PBL mirrored the fundamental values inherent in practice.

References

Barrows, H.S. & Tamblyn, R.M. (1980) *Problem-Based Learning: An Approach to Medical Education*. Springer, New York, NY.

Biley, F.C. & Smith, K.L. (1999) Making sense of problem-based learning: the perceptions and experiences of undergraduate nursing students. *Journal of Advanced Nursing*. **30**, 1205–1212.

Brookfield, S.D. (1986) *Understanding and Facilitating Adult learning: A Comprehensive Analysis of Principles and Effective Practices*. Jossey-Bass, San Francisco, CA.

Burrows, D.E. (1997) Facilitation: a concept analysis. *Journal of Advanced Nursing*. **25**, 396–404.

Carnall, L. (1998) Developing student autonomy in education: the independent option. *British Journal of Occupational Therapy*. **61** (12), 551–555.

Clouston, T.J. (2005) Facilitating tutorials in problem based learning: a students' perspective. In: *Enhancing Teaching in Higher Education - New approaches to Improving Student Learning* (eds P. Hartley *et al*.), pp. 54–64. Routledge, London.

Cornwall, M. (1998) Putting it into practice: promoting independent learning in a traditional institution. In: *Developing Student Autonomy in Learning* (ed. D. Boud), 2nd edn. pp. 242–257. Kogan Page, London.

Creedy, D. & Alavi, C. (1997) Problem-based learning in an integrated nursing curriculum. In: *The Challenge of Problem-Based Learning* (eds D. Boud & G. Feletti), 2nd edn. pp. 218–224. Kogan Page, London.

Finlay, L. (1998) *The Life World of the Occupational Therapist: Meaning and Motive in an Uncertain World*. PhD thesis, The Open University.

Glen, S. (1995) Towards a new model of nursing education. *Nurse Education Today*. **15**, 90–95.

Habermas, J. (1989) *The Theory of Communicative Action*, Vol. 2. Polity, Cambridge.

Haith-Cooper, M. (2000) Problem-based learning within health professional education. What is the role of the lecturer? A review of the literature. *Nurse Education Today*. **20**, 267–272.

Higgs, J. & Titchen, A. (1995) Propositional, professional and personal knowledge in clinical reasoning. In: *Clinical Reasoning in the Health Professions* (eds J. Higgs & M. Jones), pp. 129–146. Butterworth-Heinemann, Oxford.

Jarvis, P. (1987) *Adult Learning in the Social Context*. Croom Helm, London.

Norman, G.R. & Schmidt, H.G. (1992) The psychological basis of problem-based learning: a review of the evidence. *Academic Medicine*. **67**, 557–565.

Rolfe, G. (1998) *Expanding Nursing Knowledge: Understanding and Researching your own Practice*. Butterworth Heinemann, Oxford.

Ryan, G. (1993) Student perceptions about self-directed learning in a professional course implementing problem-based learning. *Studies in Higher Education*. **18** (1), 53–63.

Ryan, G. (1997) Ensuring that students develop an adequate and well-structured, knowledge base. In: *The Challenge of Problem-Based Learning* (eds D. Boud & G. Feletti), 2nd edn. pp. 125–136. Kogan Page, London.

Savin-Baden, M. (1997) Problem-based learning, part 2: understanding learner stances. *British Journal of Occupational Therapy*. **60** (12), 531–536.

Savin-Baden, M. (2000) *Problem-based Learning in Higher Education: Untold Stories*. SRHE and Open University Press, Buckingham.

Taylor, I. & Burgess, H. (1997) Responding to 'non-traditional' students: an enquiry and action aApproach. In: *The Challenge of Problem-Based Learning* (eds D. Boud & G. Feletti), 2nd edn. pp. 103–116. Kogan Page, London.

Titchen, A. & Higgs, J. (2001) A dynamic framework for the enhancement of health professional practice in an uncertain world: the practice knowledge interface. In: *A Practice Knowledge and Expertise in the Health Professions* (eds J. Higgs & A. Titchen), pp. 215–225. Butterworth Heinemann, Oxford.

Walker, R. (2001) Social and cultural perspectives on professional knowledge and expertise. In: *A Practice Knowledge and Expertise in the Health Professions* (eds J. Higgs & J.A. Titchen), pp. 22–28. Butterworth Heinemann, Oxford.

Weil, S. (1989) Access: towards education or miseducation? Adults imagine the future. In: *Access and Institutional Change* (ed. O. Fulton), pp. 110–143. SRHE and Open University Press, Buckingham.

14: Becoming lifelong learners in health and social care

Pam Stead, Gareth Morgan and Sally Scott-Roberts

Introduction

This chapter considers the context of lifelong learning and the impact it has on the education of professionals in health and social care. It examines the role that problem-based learning (PBL) has in the development of self-directed learners and considers a variety of potential methods that can be used to prepare them for effective lifelong learning.

What is lifelong learning?

The term is deceptively simple at face value – learning that continues over a lifetime (Field, 2000). The implications are clearly desirable for individuals, educational institutions and the workplace. There is, however, a political subtext to lifelong learning, which recognises the need for a flexible workforce, able to adapt to future changes in working practices and the demands of a modern society. This has made the definition of lifelong learning more complex, as it forms part of the discourse of both the political and economic arenas.

Lifelong learning links education to everyday life, a bridge between learning and the outside world that can empower individuals to become active, motivated learners, who are keen to improve and develop. Preparing students for lifelong learning is now an educational reality, but the challenge is how to make our educational programmes achieve this goal, which requires careful consideration of the whole process.

Why this emphasis on lifelong learning?

In the late twentieth and early twenty-first century, economic, cultural, technological and demographic changes have led governments across the developed world to introduce policies that aim to nurture a 'learning society'. In this context, the concept of lifelong learning developed as a means of ensuring personal growth and building a flexible workforce that could work creatively and collaboratively to respond to change and uncertainty.

The importance of lifelong learning has become widely recognised to empower citizens and strengthen social cohesion, with educational organisations playing their part in the preparation of learners. In higher education in United Kingdom, following the publication of the Dearing report (1997), there is an increasing expectation that education will respond to the needs of students and employers.

The health and social care focus

An increase in life expectancy in the Western world and continuous expansions in technology have led to growing expectations of health and social care services, placing often unprecedented demands on the workforce. As a consequence, professionals must keep up with the complex process of change, assimilate new knowledge and prove their ability to continually develop. They are now expected to make their practice overt and open to scrutiny. Evidence-based practice and continuing professional development has become a new focus for those working across education, health and social care and lifelong learning is a key component.

Lifelong learning therefore, has two key principles: not only for individuals to learn techniques and skills for securing employment in postmodern society, but also to enable learners to achieve their fullest potential in a rapidly changing environment. What seems to be inviolable is that professionals who demonstrate lifelong learning can respond more effectively to organisational change, which in turn has a positive impact on their clients. What, however, is less clear is how this aim can be realised. There are always different routes to achieving any long-term goal, but we believe PBL is a strong contender for being the approach of choice for its potential role in lifelong learning.

The links to problem-based learning

A socio-cultural view of education recognises the transient nature of knowledge, seeing it as susceptible to change in a fast-paced world. In health and social care settings, the current organisational and professional emphasis on evidence-based practice and lifelong learning means that learners require the skills to continually learn, acquire new knowledge and apply it to develop new ways of working. Professional education has an obligation to prepare students for the ambiguities that are the reality of practice and as a consequence, adopt a dynamic approach to knowledge and learning. This must allow them opportunity to combine what Vygotsky (1978) called scientific concepts – the theory of the discipline – with the everyday experiences of the individual (Davydov & Markova, 1983). PBL fosters this combination by acknowledging previously acquired learning, together with the specific professional knowledge needed to solve the problem presented. Because PBL uses small groups for teaching, each student's different experience can be used effectively in a group situation to broaden the knowledge of the whole group.

PBL, as a tool for the enhancement of lifelong learning, has been documented historically (Miflin *et al.*, 2000). Indeed, much of the credibility of PBL as a learning approach arguably rests on this ability. Blumberg and Michael's (1992) research suggests that the skills needed to be self-directed are enhanced by problem-based curricula. Dolmans and Schmidt (1996) claim that data from library circulation statistics demonstrate that PBL students access more material than students from a conventional curriculum; they then make the link between PBL and its impact following graduation on self-direction and see lifelong learning as an essential by-product of the PBL process.

Hmelo-Silver (2004, p. 253) cites several studies which provide

> evidence that students in PBL learn problem-solving and reasoning strategies that are transferable to new problems.

Morrison (2004) connects PBL with an enhancement of the learner's intrinsic interest in their subject and in self-directed learning skills which may persist throughout their careers. However, it has to be acknowledged that the research base connecting lifelong learning and PBL is relatively limited. Nevertheless, its ability to deliver lifelong learning can perhaps come from analysing its component attributes and making connections with its role in the *potential* for lifelong learning. Boud (1988, p. 21) points out that

> ... if students are denied opportunities to participate in decision-making about their learning, they are less likely to develop the skills they need in order to plan and organise for life-long learning ...

It seems reasonable to assume that giving students opportunities to develop these skills will enhance lifelong learning in the future.

Using PBL to promote lifelong learning

It is important that any PBL programme embeds and intrinsically supports those important skills for lifelong learning that Candy *et al.* (1994) suggest: self-directed learning, experiential learning and reflective practice. These three skills resonate with Eraut's (1994) components of professional knowledge: propositional knowledge about facts and theories, procedural knowledge about how to use and apply knowledge in the professional context and personal knowledge of oneself as a professional practitioner. Eraut's (1994) dissection of various knowledge types used by professionals is more complex than this, but these areas form a useful baseline for professional education.

A strongly student-centred ethos, utilising Roger's (1969) advocacy of active learning and Knowles (1984) principles of andragogy, is essential in recognising the particular needs and strengths of adult learners, who are motivated to learn when the subject is meaningful to them. All these are fundamental to PBL.

Motivation is integral to lifelong learning, and one of the great strengths of PBL lies in its use of realistic and challenging case studies that motivate students by immediately engaging them in the reality of practice in their chosen field. They can see the relevance of the learning to their professional career. Motivation in order to sustain lifelong learning needs to be *intrinsic* – that is, from within the person, for their own satisfaction, rather than *extrinsic*, from the need to pass exams or assignments.

These seem to us to be the key factors in contributing to satisfactory problem-solving and lifelong learning in health and social care:

▪ Overall curriculum design
▪ Self-directed learning
▪ Identifying learning needs
▪ Skills for team membership
▪ Reflective practice
▪ Professional development portfolio
▪ Practice-based learning

Overall curriculum design

In order for the intended outcome of lifelong learning to occur, it is essential that the whole curriculum, including methods of assessment, is geared to support and encourage learners to take control of their own learning. An important part of the ability to be cohesive in this approach is the wholehearted support of staff, which means new teaching staff have to be supported in their introduction to PBL and have opportunity to develop their skills with a more experienced colleague. Peer reflection and discussion between staff that teach parallel groups is key to staff development.

Support is essential not just for those who teach within the programme but also practitioners who provide placements for students from PBL courses. It takes time and support for learners from more traditional educational backgrounds to adjust to PBL. In the same way, it requires support from the programme to assist practitioners to understand how PBL works in order for them to facilitate student learning on placement.

PBL offers a framework that fosters joint initial problem identification, negotiated learning goals that guide individual research, as well as informed problem-solving (Barrows & Tamblyn, 1980). This context of a united programme gives the basis for PBL to have lifelong learning as a natural outcome. We describe the key components of the PBL framework that contribute to life-long learning.

Self-directed learning

An important issue is the development of independent research skills. We use the term *research* here to mean the ability to independently find out information. Students come with varying levels of skill, depending on their background. The availability of good learning resources is crucial to a successful PBL programme, and support to effectively utilise these resources is equally important. For instance, students require time to gain research skills and sufficient support from library staff from the outset of their studies.

Self-directed learning is necessary for the students to gain the propositional knowledge required for understanding and working with the case study. These are the facts and the theoretical underpinnings needed to address the case study. These research skills are by no means the only component of self-directed learning. Students have to learn to identify what it is that they need to research and have an understanding of why that research is thought to be necessary for the case study, and this should be elicited by the group discussion, supported by the tutor.

The motivation of learners to be self-directed is essential to this process. What is clear is that the ability to be self-directed is multifactorial and the expectation on students to self-direct is not confined to propositional knowledge – they are learning about the process of learning (see Taylor, 1997, for quotes from her students which illustrate this). Savin-Baden (2000) refers to students exploring and creating knowledge, and it is these process skills that are so vital to lifelong learning.

Using PBL in this way, students are developing the skills for lifelong learning, improving various strategies to assist their learning, whilst building a sense of self-efficacy that gives the confidence to be self-directed.

Identifying learning needs

The topic of selecting and designing material that is relevant for case studies is discussed elsewhere in this book, so presupposing suitable triggers for PBL, when working with a case study, the group has to identify the learning needs that arise from it. These relate not just to the group's need to investigate aspects of the case study but they also link to the learning needs of the individuals in the group. The learning needs and how they are going to be met are, in our experience, best written using a learning contract. The group members each identify what they need to find out and how they are going to do it. They then research their agreed topic and report back to the group. This is a cyclical process, not only within a case study, but the process will be repeated throughout the programme as the students work with a variety of different triggers. It is important that students learn to identify for themselves the gaps in their knowledge and decide how they can resolve them.

Tutor support is essential in the early stages, to help students appraise the quality and depth of their research though this support is reduced as the course progresses and students learn how to critique their own and each other's research. The role of the tutor is essentially as a facilitator to help the group monitor its own learning (see Chapter 5 for more discussion on facilitation).

It is important to realise that research and suggestions are appraised and discussed increasingly in terms of their relevance to the case study. In this way, students on health-care programmes learn to clinically reason as they justify why they have selected a particular assessment tool or an intervention method for a case study. Also integral to this process is the examination of other possibilities, which may be discarded. This justification process is essential to the development of the group's learning. Recent legislation has reinforced the need for practitioners to remain accountable for their practice, so rehearsal of these justification processes also helps prepare students for practice. Service users are entitled to explicit, evidenced-based decisions, which reflect well-developed clinical reasoning, and this is best nurtured in the relatively supportive atmosphere of a PBL group before students have to deal with multidisciplinary teams and vulnerable clients.

PBL was found by Mattingly and Fleming (1994) to develop clinical reasoning more quickly than traditional learning. The nature of PBL requires participants to take ownership of the problem and ultimately the learning. All participants in the group have a part to play in reaching a consensus about how to deal with problems presented, and in doing so, will uncover knowledge about their own preferred learning styles.

The need to share acquired applied knowledge with peers, and then later in practice with colleagues, demands a process of overt reasoning, but also places a responsibility on the individual to adopt a range of communication skills that are efficient and fit for purpose and audience. A number of studies have identified that PBL students have reported their continuing ability to integrate and apply knowledge aptly to enhance their decision-making (Davys & Pope, 2006). The link to lifelong learning is clear. Students who are able to identify their own learning needs on a regular basis and are used to finding out how to meet those needs are going to be better situated for future independent learning.

Skills for team membership

If we consider lifelong learning to encompass personal as well as professional development, another important impact of PBL is its effect on interpersonal skills. In striving to improve the efficiency and effectiveness of health and social care, there has been recognition that joined-up working is necessary. Multidisciplinary teamwork requires practitioners from different disciplines to share profession-specific knowledge in an endeavour to negotiate solutions to increasingly complex problems. Successful, shared decision-making requires practitioners to adopt group processes, which are fostered by PBL (Salvatori, 2000; Davys & Pope, 2006).

In PBL, students learn to communicate effectively in groups, taking it in turns to assume the role of group leader. Students are encouraged to resolve issues that arise within the group themselves, as far as possible, in order to develop the ability to work in teams. Being able to understand other worker's perspectives is an important aspect of teamwork (Fenwick, 2002) and discussions within the groups soon make learners realise their viewpoint is not always universally shared. There is no doubt that conflict will be experienced at some point but sharing different views with the same goal in mind gives the opportunity for working compromises, which reflects the reality of multidisciplinary team working in health and social care. Savin-Baden (2000) makes the point that these skills are highly valued in the labour market and PBL provides an opportunity for students to learn these skills in an integrated way in the context of a real-life case study.

Reflective practice

The unique nature of the problems presented by the individual often demands tailor-made solutions. These cannot rely on textbook answers and requires reasoning that incorporates evaluation of knowledge and learning. Schön (1987) suggests that this can be achieved through a process of conscious contemplation, in other words reflection. Chapter 8 offers a more detailed discussion on reflection, but it is important to emphasise here that reflection allows practice to be evaluated and questioned.

PBL requires students to reflect not only upon their learning but upon the processes they adopt in problem-solving, in effect, their own clinical reasoning. This ensures that knowledge, in the widest sense of the term, remains explicit and open for evaluation. It is only in questioning and evaluating that practice can be improved and developed.

Reflection, like most other skills, requires practice and, if introduced prior to professional registration, can equip new practitioners with opportunities to have engaged, practiced and evaluated its role in their own professional development.

For some professionals, lifelong learning is evidenced formally by continuous professional development (CPD). This has been identified as the 'ongoing progression in knowledge, thinking and skills development' that all professional and some support workers are now expected to engage with (Westcott, 2005, p. 88).

CPD is now a requirement for maintenance of professional registration for allied health professionals. It has become apparent that higher education institutions preparing professionals to enter the workforce now have an increased responsibility to prepare them for this new era and to equip them with the skills to maintain their CPD portfolio.

Professional development portfolio

The portfolio is probably the most tangible indication any student can have of the professional requirement for lifelong learning and it is, in our view, essential to integrate a professional portfolio into the programme from the beginning. It can then be added to and developed to show the student's progress to themselves, the faculty and to future employers. It becomes a learning resource and establishes early in the student's career the importance of regular monitoring and reflection on their learning. The portfolio contains a distillation of the student's reflections on their various experiences during the course. Reflective practice is seen as playing a pivotal role in the development of competent professionals and essential to lifelong learning (Schön, 1983). Students should be encouraged to reflect not only on significant learning events for their portfolio, but also on their group work and their own personal development, as a regular feature in the programme.

Knowledge of self is key in professional practice (Eraut, 1994). Propositional knowledge and procedural knowledge can be gained and recorded relatively easily in a professional portfolio, whereas self-knowledge is only revealed by reflective practice (Fish & Twinn, 1997). The veracity of any documentation of professional reflective practice is debatable, though superficial reflection of personal practice is not difficult to identify. We have found that a personal tutor system helps support the reflective process.

Practice-based learning and PBL

Practice-based learning (clinical fieldwork practice) is essential to professional development in health and social care, and forms a large part of any professional programme. Experiential learning from practice is recognised as integral and time spent in developing and supporting practice educators is invaluable, not just giving them information about the programme and the procedures involved in taking and assessing a student but also a theoretical underpinning of the foundations of modern educational practice and PBL.

We strongly take the view that practice educators form part of the wider teaching team and that they have a right (and a duty) to learn about PBL in order to be able to provide a consistent approach when the students are with them on placement. Practitioners who do not understand PBL can be injurious to student's self-esteem and confidence, so it is essential that practice educators are equally committed to the principles of PBL, and that they are supported in their own educational development.

Practice-based learning makes a significant contribution to the PBL groups back in the university, forming a large part of the students' procedural knowledge. Following placement, students are able to utilise this experiential knowledge base to refine their clinical reasoning, and the integration of different experiences adds to the rich mix of discussions and justifications for a variety of interventions. Use and integration of practice learning in this way is designed to help break down any differences the students see between theory and practice. Evaluation of practice is essential to professional development and sets the scene for continuation of the process after graduation.

Integration of practice into education in this way provides many advantages, not least being the important role in maintaining motivation for students who can start to visualise themselves moving closer to their professional goal. Students are encouraged to imagine themselves as future educators, sustaining a link with education and future professional development.

Conclusion

This chapter started by justifying the need for lifelong learning in health and social care and then has made the case for PBL to be used to help budding professionals achieve that aim. We have described the key elements needed to design a programme that supports lifelong learning and shown that the processes developed, modified and evaluated during PBL foster practices that are necessary to modern day professionals, as inevitable changes in health and social care require practitioners to maintain a lifelong learning perspective. PBL is not the only way for students to develop such a perspective but it does provide a sound base for the development of the necessary knowledge, skills and attitudes for lifelong learning.

References

Barrows, H. & Tamblyn, R. (1980) *Problem–Based Learning: An Approach to Medical Education*. Springer Publishing Company, New York, NY.

Blumberg, P. & Michael, J.A. (1992) The development of self-directed behaviours in a partially teacher-directed problem-based learning curriculum. *Teaching and Learning in Medicine.* **4** (1), 3–8.

Boud, D. (1988) *Developing Student Autonomy in Learning*, 2nd edn. Kogan Page, London.

Candy, P., Crebert, G. & O'Leary, J. (1994) *Developing lifelong learners through undergraduate education.* Australian Government Publishing Service, Canberra.

Davydov, V.V. & Markova, A.A. (1983) A concept of educational activity for school children. *Soviet Psychology.* **2** (2), 50–76.

Davys, D. & Pope, K. (2006) Problem-based learning within occupational therapy education: a summary of the Salford experience. *British Journal of Occupational Therapy.* **69** (12), 572–574.

Dearing, R. (1997) *Summary report of the UK Committee of Inquiry into HE: higher education in the learning society.* HMSO, London.

Dolmans, D. & Schmidt, H. (1996) The advantages of problem-based curricula. *Postgraduate Medical Journal.* **72**, 535–538.

Eraut, M. (1994) *Developing Professional Knowledge and Competence.* Falmer Press, London.

Fenwick, T.J. (2002) Problem-based learning, group process and the mid-career professional: implications for graduate education. *Higher Education Research and Development.* **21** (1), 5–21.

Field, J. (2000) *Lifelong Learning and the New Educational Order.* Trentham Books, Stoke on Trent.

Fish, D. & Twinn, S. (1997). *Quality Clinical Supervision in the Healthcare Professions.* Butterworth-Heinemann, Oxford.

Hmelo-Silver, C.E. (2004) Problem–based learning: what and how do students learn? *Educational Psychology Review.* **16** (3), 235–265.

Knowles, M.S (1984) *Andragogy in Action.* Jossey Bass, San Francisco, CA.

Mattingly, C. & Fleming, M.H. (1994) *Clinical Reasoning: Forms of Enquiry in Therapeutic Practice.* FA Davis Co, Philadelphia, PA.

Miflin, B.M., Campbell, C.B. & Price, D.A (2000) A conceptual framework to guide the development of self-directed, life long learning in problem-based medical curricula. *Medical Education.* **34** (4), 299–306.

Morrison, J. (2004) Where now for problem based learning? *The Lancet.* **363** (1), 174.

Salvatori, P. (2000) Implementing a problem-based curriculum in occupational therapy: a conceptual model. *Australian Journal of Occupational Therapy.* **47** (3), 119–133.

Savin-Baden, M. (2000). *Problem Based Learning in Higher Education: Untold Stories.* The Society for Research into Higher Education and Open University Press, Buckingham.

Schön, D.A. (1983) *The Reflective Practitioner: How Professionals Think in Action.* Temple Smith, London.

Schön, D.A. (1987) *Educating the Reflective Practitioner: Toward a New Design for Teaching and Learning in the Professions.* Jossey Bass, San Francisco, CA.

Taylor, I. (1997) *Developing Learning in Professional Education: Partnerships for Practice*. The Society for Research into Higher Education and Open University Press, Buckingham.

Vygotsky, L.S. (1978) *Mind in Society: The Development of Higher Psychological Processes*. Harvard University Press, Cambridge, MA.

Westcott, L. (2005) Continuing professional development. In: *Working in Health and Social Care: An Introduction for Allied Health Professionals* (eds T. Clouston & L. Westcott), pp. 87–102. Elsevier/Churchill Livingstone, Edinburgh.

15: Becoming a self-directed learner

Susan Delport and Ruth Squire

Introduction

This chapter aims to set out and define self-directed learning within the context of professional education for health and social care. Initially, the idea of becoming a self-directed learner will be examined in relation to an overall educational philosophy of student centredness, in particular, problem-based learning (PBL). PBL in this context is taken to mean a method of delivery of teaching which in part enables small groups of students to explore triggers like case studies or scenarios. This is done by identifying issues that need to be researched, carrying out that research and then sharing and discussing together the knowledge gained within the group in order to develop solutions. Links will be made between self-directed learning and becoming a lifelong learner in recognition of the recent increased importance of the latter as part of the profile of a health and social care professional.

Further discussion will take place around the expectations of both students and tutors on a PBL programme, as to the quality and quantity of knowledge acquired while being self-directed learners. We will explore the process of becoming a self-directed learner and illustrate how various tools and resources can assist or act as a barrier to this learning. This will be followed by an acknowledgement of the intra- and interpersonal skills and qualities of individual students and tutors in the learning process, examining for example, how confidence and motivation can impact the ability to develop as a self-directed learner.

We will then go onto uncover some of the challenges of being and becoming a self-directed learner from both the students and tutors' perspectives, including some of the challenges faced. The authors' ultimate goal is to share with the reader their practical ideas and collective experiences on how to overcome many of these issues. Finally, a summary of the key elements for developing the skills of self-directed learning will be provided, highlighting the benefits of this educational philosophy which we believe can be applied to any educational programme for health or social care professionals.

What is a self-directed learner?

First, let us tackle the issue of terminology. The use of the terms *student-directed learner* and *self-directed learner* appear to be interchangeable within the literature and convey the same meaning. One of the goals for students within a health and social care context is to become a practitioner who is also a lifelong self-directed learner. Therefore, for the purposes of this chapter, the authors have chosen to refer to self-directed learners.

Knowles (1975, p. 18) describes self-directed learning as

> a process in which individuals take the initiative, with or without the help of others, in diagnosing their learning needs, formulating learning goals, identifying human and material resources for learning, choosing and implementing appropriate learning strategies, and evaluating learning outcomes.

This encapsulates the ethos of a positive student experience in a PBL curriculum.

Long (2000) asserts that in order to sustain self-directed learning, students need

▪ confidence;
▪ a certain level of competence;
▪ control to make choices.

Long (2005) distinguishes between different perceptions of self-directed learning and discusses both independent learning, where the learners are on their own and only accountable to themselves, and distance learning. In distance learning, the student is geographically separated from their teacher and with a pre-set curriculum; importantly however, the learner has some choices and psychological control over how they will learn. This is a key distinction because it is the learners' attitude of assuming control of the learning that signifies self-direction. Whilst not engaged in distance learning, self-direction in this sense is vital in PBL as much of the learning occurs through the medium of group work and tutorials. Students are therefore not self-directed in terms of the definition above of the autonomous independent learner, yet they still assume psychological control in deciding how and what they will investigate to fully explore the issue at hand. It is this psychological control that we are referring to in terms of being self-directed within a PBL course.

Self-directed learning fits comfortably within the educational philosophy of student-centred learning. This style of learning is one in which the students are active participants (Clouston, 2005), are responsible for determining their own learning needs and for evaluating the success in meeting those needs. There is a shift in balance of power between the tutor and the student, compared to traditional didactic programmes of study. It is therefore plain how fostering self-directed learning fits philosophically within a student-centred curriculum.

How can we identify a self-directed learner?

Burns (1995) postulates that by the time we reach adulthood, we are all self-directed, arguing that this humanistic approach to adult learning should incorporate elements of a student centredness, turning the whole andragogical experience back onto the student. Andragogy in this instance refers to adult learning. Indeed Bhat et al. (2007, p. 1) noted that the action of being self-directed is a 'purposive mental process' involving a development of continuous goal setting and decision making for which the students must accept responsibility (Long, 2005).

As PBL occurs mostly in small groups, students need to work cooperatively with others. Their participation in these groups has been linked to their acceptance of self-directed learning (Clouston, 2007). Being cognisant of students' contribution in the group may therefore be a useful tool for facilitators to determine learners' ability to direct their own learning. This said, it is also acknowledged that learning takes many forms, and some students may play a greater role outside of the group context to this end.

We already know from much educational research that internal motivation is a key intrapersonal factor in the process of learning (Entwistle, 1998; Dolmans et al., 2005; Hall & Moseley, 2005). In addition to this, Childs (2005) found that students who had an internal locus of control (i.e. attributed success or failure to factors within themselves), were more likely to be motivated by self-directed learning.

Fazey and Fazey (2001) suggest that research has shown that autonomous individuals are indicative of achievement and such individuals often demonstrate achievement behaviours of diligence, curiosity, flexibility towards failure and dedication towards progress (see also Harter, 1990; Bandura, 1997). For staff, it may be possible to identify these individuals at an early stage, perhaps even on admission into higher education with suitable selection processes.

Educationalists generally favour deep learning that is retained and drawn upon over a prolonged timescale, rather than a surface learning approach where facts are easily forgotten beyond the short term (typified by last minute cramming for an examination). This is because surface learning often means information is assimilated without an understanding of the concepts, or becomes strategic and assessment driven (Ramsden, 1992; Biggs, 2003). What is important here is that deep learning is more likely to occur when a student is self-directed. Whilst readers may be familiar with features of deep learning, it may be useful to recap some key aspects. Active learning, interacting with others and relating new ideas to existing knowledge are all characteristics required of students if they are to acquire a deeper level of understanding. Long (2005) notes that these processes are enjoyable for students and this helps in linking the task to past experiences, thus further facilitating deep learning. Parnell (2001) suggests that students who start to reflect on their thinking processes are demonstrating they can take responsibility for their own learning, and are therefore engaging in deep learning (Chapter 8).

In addition to this is the idea of context. Biggs (2003) highlighted that one of the main ways to encourage deep learning is to provide good motivational context for the students. For health or social care students, this translates into devising a series of real-life scenarios for study which link together, building up their professional education and helping to shape students into potential nurses, social workers or physiotherapists to name but a few.

As well as having the internal motivational context and complex interpersonal skills mentioned above, the self-directed learners also need to possess the practical ability to go off on their own and gather relevant literature from suitable academic sources. This requires technical knowledge and confidence in utilising a range of resources, for example university libraries and appropriate sites on the internet. Other helpful attributes of the self-directed learner include organisational ability and efficient information processing, being able to filter out vast amounts of irrelevant information and select the useful and relevant sources.

It is apparent that some new undergraduates may not be fully prepared for these demanding challenges and therefore any student-centred programme needs to facilitate the development of these skills. Some practicalities of how an educational programme is designed and the ways in which tutors can assist in this development, will be discussed in more depth later (see also Chapter 4).

Expectations of self-directed learning

Wider context of expectations

Before considering the specific expectations of student learners within a PBL course, it is important to consider the context and goal of the learning, as these form both the basis and rationale for facilitating a self-directed approach. The ultimate goal for both tutors and students on any health or social care programme (like radiography or medicine), is for students to achieve a degree that enables each person to practice competently within a particular professional context. To ensure that individuals graduating from these courses throughout the United Kingdom are fit to practice, awarding programmes are required to comply with the minimum standards of relevant professional and regulatory bodies.

This creates potential conflict within a self-directed philosophy of learning. There is a situation where the curriculum content is prescribed by professional requirements and the end product is determined by these set standards, yet the learner wishes to choose the process of their own learning (Brookfield, 1986). Those who participate in the learning can however shape the programme to some extent. The unique nature of courses within health and social care is that students are preparing to deal with individuals in need. As health and social care professionals, they will need to apply an ever increasing and changing body of knowledge to real-life situations.

As knowledge and technology expand, health and social care programmes can no longer cover all that needs to be learnt, and neither can they predict what changes might occur (Fischer, 2000). Lifelong learning has been advocated as a way of keeping abreast of current developments in health and social care to ensure that clients receive the best possible care (Chapter 14). One of the key skills of lifelong learning is the ability to be self-directed. Clinical instructors of physical therapy students recognised that self-directed learning was one of the seven attributes that illustrated students' ability to practice at entry level (Jette *et al.*, 2007). This attribute also needs to move way beyond this point, as careers can extend more than 40 years for some new practitioners. Professionals therefore will need to develop self-directed learning to keep abreast of developments in their fields of work.

The expectations of students on becoming a self-directed learner

It is important that students enrolling on a PBL course are made aware from the start that self-directed learning will be an essential part of the programme. Given the importance of intrinsic motivation for a major programme of study, ensuring a student group enrols with a commitment to a self-directed learning will enhance the experience right from the start. Sending potential students information about the course and crucially explaining the method of learning and teaching prior to interview, is one way to make expectations clear. If possible, the interview process can reflect these expectations and allow students an experience to typify the course that they are applying for. This can be modelled, say, within a mock tutorial group at interview, where a group of applicants discuss their understanding of a topic that they have been asked to prepare beforehand (like their understanding of the chosen profession). In the session, they can share their learning and be encouraged to identify aspects they would identify for further research. Such methods make clear to candidates, in a very practical way, the expectation of independent study. A further exploration of the candidate's ability to work independently and take responsibility for their own learning can then be explored during individual interviews. In theory, the potential student is made aware that being self-directed will be an important part of a PBL curriculum.

It is important to note however, that each student begins from a different starting point. Some students can come directly from secondary education where little autonomy and self-direction was required for success. Whilst they are aware that self-directed learning is part of a PBL course, they may struggle to acquire the new skills required to be in control of their own learning. In contrast, by choosing to study later in life, some mature students have already demonstrated self-direction in relation to their learning. They may also face challenges embarking on the road to becoming self-directed, particularly in their academic confidence. It is important to recognise from the outset that both past and present experiences of all students should be valued for a more holistic learning experience (Bonello, 2001).

Some students may be reluctant self-directed learners (Knowles, 1975). It takes more effort and time to take control of your learning. Students may arrive with expectations that tutors will provide expertise and be the source of knowledge. It can be a painful process for students to rely on their own ability to seek knowledge from a range of sources, have faith in this ability and belief in their analytical skills to know what is sufficient. Students can struggle in deciding what level of knowledge is needed to comprehend the phenomena under study, and the transition to self-directed learning can be a traumatic experience (Mazhindu, 1990). Some students feel more comfortable and safe with a more ordered and structured model of learning and teaching (Nolan & Nolan, 1997), highlighting the importance of clarity when recruiting to a PBL course. Students have different life experiences, personalities and different styles of learning. Staff need to be aware of this to understand how these factors impact on students' ability to take control of their learning.

Students expect tutors to be responsive and obliging, along with having the ability to restore their self-confidence (Childs, 2005). This is linked to anxiety about self-directed learning, especially if they have not had previous experience of this style of learning. Whilst support should be available throughout a programme, tutors need to be particularly approachable to first-year students who have to learn and practice new skills. Childs (2005) reports that students are concerned that they might not get the support they need, but that they are willing to approach tutors themselves to use them as a resource if needed. It is helpful if the programme recognises the necessity of support and provides an explicit system to help students develop the skills they need in line with the expectations made of them.

Expectations of tutors

In PBL, tutors expect students to be proactive in developing the skills needed to take control of their learning. It is acknowledged that becoming a self-directed learner is a developmental process, albeit an important one for the progression of professional development linked to lifelong learning. Tutors should be aware that students have a wide range of abilities and life experiences, and that their learning needs will be unique and specific. Although students' learning styles may differ, as part of the expectation for self-directed learning, tutors might usefully anticipate that students can identify and explore the implications of their personal learning style. From this point, they can then make suggestions about how to best meet that student's needs within the learning required. Students are expected to contribute to the group from their life experiences (Knowles, 1975), and this linkage will enhance both their learning and that of their peers. The contributions of students are seen as being equally valuable as those of tutors.

One of the fundamental principles of self-directed learning is that students need time to choose the resources and methods appropriate to meet their identified learning needs. To help this process, tutors are advised to set aside clearly identified slots within the timetabled week that allow the students to pursue their individual learning. This sets an expectation that students should use this type of time to research the given topic, and problems arise if this does not occur. We will discuss this later as one of the challenges facing tutors.

Skills and resources needed for self-directed learning

As stated previously, self-directed learning is a developmental process. Some students come with a readiness to learn in this way; others develop the skills over time. The theory of readiness to learn within a PBL style has already been discussed in depth in Chapter 3. We will now consider here a range of skills that students will need to learn in order to thrive within this student-centred philosophy of learning. Academically, some students might need more support to develop the cognitive skills required to investigate, collate, analyse and synthesise vast quantities of reading material (Bhat *et al.*, 2007). Tutors will need to ensure that they create environments that cultivate the development of these abilities. Below are a range of skills and practical considerations to assist students to become effective self-directed learners. These skills have been grouped into intrapersonal, interpersonal and process skills.

Intrapersonal attributes

For use in this context, intrapersonal skills refer to skills necessary for individuals to develop within themselves.

Coping with anxiety about this novel way of working

For some students, the perceived lack of structure imposed by the staff or an authority figure can create a sense of unease and lack of confidence in the content, quality and direction of the programme. Students can become concerned if emphasis moves away from the end product, for example, onto group process. Students need to have a clear understanding of the PBL system, and staff teams can help this through their supportive documentation for students. It is also helpful if students are assured that their programme has met the criteria of quality regulators like the Quality Assurance Agency (QAA, 2001). Students can doubt initially whether they are learning sufficiently, but experience into the curriculum often leads to considerable skills in tracking their own growth and development through professional development tutorials and tools such as a continuing professional development (CPD) portfolio.

Confidence and belief in self

Fazey and Fazey (2001) argue that if individuals have confidence in their own ability and academic competence, they are more likely to take responsibility for and be comfortable with self-directed learning. One of the key roles for the facilitator (and the rest of the group) is to support and acknowledge each student's contribution to boost their self-confidence and perception of their competence. Constructive and appropriate feedback is a vital part of this process.

Self-evaluation

Childs (2005) found that this was one area that students found difficult and were often unsure about the quality of their work. The students with an internal locus of control tended to equate their marks with the effort and time expended, and were surprised when their marks did not reflect that. To avoid self-evaluation being linked solely to marks gained, students need to be supported to achieve their learning outcomes in alternative ways with additional strategies (Childs, 2005).

Group evaluation can be encouraged in PBL, both in terms of the process (contribution to the group) and in terms of product (handout/presentation produced). This can help individual students to further reflect and self-evaluate, enabling behavioural change. Long (2005) has reflected that self-evaluation goes alongside an ability to be self-aware. In this way, self-evaluation yields substance and tangible evidence beyond the amount of effort exerted. Students need to know where their strengths lie, but also their limitations. They need to know how they learn best and what hinders this. With heightened self-awareness, comes the ability to seek help when it is appropriate, and thereby optimise learning.

Interpersonal skills

These skills are needed to be self-directed within a PBL course. Without them, students become limited in their ability to tap into the range of resources available.

Knowing when to ask for help and support and how to utilise a range of resources

Some students struggle to own this responsibility and lack confidence to ask for help, whilst others turn to tutors but still do not think of asking other useful people like fellow students or practitioners. Students need to be encouraged to widen their horizons to the vast sea of information that is available from a full range of sources.

Ability to facilitate other adults' ability to grow and develop

The concept of working collaboratively in groups reflects the team ethos in which most health and social care professionals function. Facilitating trust and mutual support does not necessarily happen automatically. By working in groups, students learn the skills of fostering growth and development in their peers (Clouston & Whitcombe, 2005). They also learn to trust the work of others and how to depend professionally on the contribution of others. Childs (2005) reports that students frequently used their peer group to assist with their self-evaluation, as well as for support. The skills of interdependence, considering others' opinions, views and knowledge, as well as giving and receiving constructive criticism are all life skills that are essential for effective health and social care practice. By developing these skills in the academic environment, student practitioners are well prepared for their professional lives.

Process skills

Cognitive, information processing and organisational skills are all required to study in a self-directed way. This section will outline some of the tools that can be applied to help develop these important skills.

Learning contracts

A learning contract is a negotiated agreement or learning plan and usefully lies at the heart of self-directed learning (Stephenson & Laycock, 1993; Whitcombe, 2001). The students are required to identify their learning needs, select the most appropriate methods and resources to achieve these and then set criteria to evaluate whether they have been met. Students can be encouraged to use a learning contract within their group work. This ensures that the group is focused and each student knows what work they will achieve, and the documentation helps ensure accountability for the work each has agreed to cover. Learning contracts can also be used within practice/clinical education to take into account previous experience and future learning needs.

Organisational and time management strategies

In order to feel in control and to maintain a sense of enjoyment in learning, students need to adopt organisational and time management strategies early on in the programme (Childs, 2005). This includes how to utilise allocated self-directed study time and how to block further periods of time to accomplish tasks set. At any one time, students may be researching information for several modules or triggers (e.g. a case study, scenarios or other concept to elicit investigation) and need to develop a clear filing/information management system from the outset to help maintain a sense of direction and focus. Students may need to ensure that they compile a clear contents page for any handouts or other resources they produce in order to return easily to this material at a later date (this would be especially useful in a spiral curriculum design – Chapter 4). Whatever system is adopted by each student, it should have meaning to that individual and is best encouraged and implemented at the beginning of the programme before the volume of content to manage feels insurmountable.

Learning how to use available resources

Practicalities such as photocopying and using library facilities, have an impact on any self-directed learner (Clouston, 2005), as it is only when students master these elements that learning can be facilitated rather than hindered. Students will need to learn how to access search engines, which ones to use and how to select appropriate words for electronic journal searches. Some can feel overwhelmed by the process of searching for information and may need initial help with a few selected website addresses or key authors. Those with little pre-existing awareness of a topic, in particular, may struggle in knowing where to start searching into a new area. This may even result in avoiding topics where students feel less competent (Long, 2005). When tutors are facilitating a working group, sharing resources or strategies for gathering information can help counter any tendency for this type of trend.

How to utilise the literature

Knowles (1975) refers to this as proactive learning, that is, not reading a book from cover to cover, but using the contents list or index to find the relevant sections to answer the questions of particular self-directed inquiry. Payne and Whittaker (2000) in their useful book on developing study skills, suggest the 'SQ3R' method of approaching reading material. This refers to first surveying the content in a general manner, developing a questioning technique of who, what, when, where and how for each section, and then finally read, recall and review the section. They assert that this method helps students to read systematically and purposefully. Childs (2005) found that some students became discouraged when they read with the intention of understanding the content, because of the length of time taken to this end. She suggests that alternative strategies such as active reading, skimming, self-testing, rereading or slowing the pace when the subject content was difficult, might contribute to a more satisfying method of collecting information. Reinforcing these types of advice in student documentation will assist learners in developing the skills they need.

Analysis and synthesis skills

These are high-level processing skills that are needed to understand, integrate and apply theory to practice. Frequently, vast quantities of reading material need to be digested to find the most useful material. At the beginning of study, students should be encouraged to use at least two or three sources of information when exploring an area. This means they can start to look at different academic views, and compare and contrast the information they gather. When students bring their information back to the group, they need to be encouraged to summarise what they have read (rather than bringing a textbook or information printed off from the internet) to explain the information gathered. This process of summary is important as it assists in developing the required analytical skills. When several students have researched the same topic, they can be encouraged to combine their information, applying this information in a holistic way to the trigger under study, especially when producing a handout, as this helps with developing synthesis skills.

How to use web-based learning environments

With such easy access to the Internet, students can work on projects together without being in the same room. At a very basic level, students are encouraged to use an Internet-based education support system such as Blackboard Academic Suite (Blackboard Inc., 1997). For many students, this is a new skill, and can be somewhat overwhelming at first, but once mastered, this type of system allows greater freedom to learn through research and debate.

Professional development portfolio

As mentioned previously, the purpose of the portfolio is to assist students, from the start, to reflect on experiences and to take control of their learning, identifying gaps and evaluating their progress (Jasper, 1995). It is good practice for students to start gathering a portfolio immediately, so they are empowered to reflect on their development as a self-directed learner within a professional context (see also Chapter 8).

Challenges to developing the skills of a self-directed learner

The students' perspective

As discussed previously, from the students' perspective, it is important they recognise and value a need for readiness in learning. Brookfield (1986) cites research carried out by Penland (1977) that linked this readiness with a student's ability to coordinate and carry through independent learning. Some students may struggle to reach this stage, in terms of their skills development, and then go on to show either a lack of engagement with the task or become strategic about what they learn (Clouston, 2005). As we know, these actions are contrary to the philosophy of deep learning and so become a real challenge within educational settings as far as both students and tutors are concerned. One solution is to try to encourage individuals to gain more insight into their level of readiness. This can be helped through one-to-one meetings with their personal tutors or other academic staff and also by engaging in greater levels of reflection.

Other challenges for the self-directed learner might arise from inadvertent overloading of students with task-driven outcomes, like presentations, producing handouts, excessive course reading lists or time spent writing too many assignments. This is of particular concern in modular programmes, especially where split assessments are used within modules. Biggs (2003) and Gibbs (1992) both warn of the dangers of heavy workloads, stressing that the outcome of this approach results in superficial learning.

So how much is too much? Achieving the right balance of all these ingredients is particularly difficult within a PBL style course as time is often a key factor to allow enough in-depth study for the individual in between group tutorials.

Another challenge often posed to courses run within PBL philosophy is that students lack basic skills or knowledge required to practice as health or social care professionals (Schmidt, 2000; Ibrahim *et al.*, 2006). It is worth noting that these authors are challenging the medical education model of PBL which differs from most health and social care models (as discussed in Chapter 2). It is not the remit here to enter into this debate, only to present the reader with how we have found this particular style to be successful for many years. Institutions can then deliberate the issues within their respective departments. This said, the challenge of quantity and/or quality of information gathering remains an issue for many students. How much information and knowledge should be attained and to what depth should this be studied? The emphasis is on the process of learning, developing strategies to use available resources and understanding concepts, rather than just learning facts.

The tutors' perspective

One of the primary challenges to any tutor new to facilitating self-directed learners is that of relinquishing control and avoiding becoming the expert who is there to impart knowledge (Jamrozik, 1996). Answering direct questions has its place in the PBL tutorial but as the reader will see from the discussion in Chapter 5 (Facilitation in PBL), there is a fine line between setting yourself up as an expert and being a good facilitator of student learning. Knowing when to be a useful resource and how to share that knowledge, takes fine judgement and sensitivity to ensure that only the questions the students have asked are answered and not the ones the tutor thinks should be answered. The challenge for tutors is to ask probing questions to stimulate students to seek answers and to harness their curiosity to research and discover for themselves, rather than to be told what the tutor thinks they need to know.

As already discussed, it is vital that initial motivation is cultivated to help individuals grow and develop their own skills. Motivation is therefore a potential challenge for tutors (Rogers, 2001). Adult learners (unlike children) are free to leave. There are many detractors from learning that can get in the way. Adult learners may experience difficulty juggling time and family commitments as well as finances. On top of this, feeling academically stretched can all drain the motivation they start out with. To maintain quality independent study and indeed to plumb the depths, takes a great deal of personal motivation. Where this is lacking, the tutor may wish to see the student and together reach consensus about the way forward. Utilising students' past experiences to build on knowledge and valuing all the learners as equals can assist motivation. The experiences held by an 18-year-old school leaver who may have lived through a close relative dying from cancer are as valued as the mature student who will have equally rich experiences from which to draw. This becomes more challenging when the mature students may appear more confident and able to express their opinions within a group setting. This said, all students may face perceptions of inadequacies about their academic competence. Facilitating both group and peer feedback can help to build confidence and motivation.

Finally, it is interesting to consider how to deal with the student who relinquishes responsibility to become self-directed. Facilitating a deep approach to learning poses a real challenge to tutors. Students who have a tendency to gloss over areas at a superficial level in order to produce an end product, will need prompting and challenging to encourage them to delve more deeply. A challenge to tutors is to know when students have mastered the basics, especially in preparation for practice experience in health and social care settings, as there is a duty of care to clients. Practitioners and clients need to have the confidence that students are competent for the level of the ensuing placement. Whilst self-directed learning is advocated, there are still clear expectations that need to be met in order to meet requirements for safe practice, and these need clear communication.

Conclusion

In summary, a self-directed learner is someone who takes responsibility for their own learning. They use a range of resources that suit their learning style to meet their learning needs, and are able to evaluate how successfully they have met the criteria for their learning. Successful PBL programmes rely on attracting students who display the attributes of self-directed learners. Combining readiness to learn, facilitating deep learning and harnessing the motivation to develop the skills of the self-directed learner within students, are challenges facing both the PBL tutors and students alike.

An individual working within an ever changing health and social care context will need to keep abreast of current evidenced-based practice, and will need the skills of self-directed learning to do so.

Some of these skills have been discussed in detail in this chapter, and include developing certain intrapersonal, interpersonal and process skills. Practical solutions have been offered and advice given to assist both students and tutors to progress along the continuum. If these skills can be fostered and nurtured at an undergraduate or pre-registration level, it will make the entry and journey into the working world a little less daunting. Being self-directed is a lifelong skill – a process rather than a product, which will continue to develop way beyond initial qualification.

References

Bandura, A. (1997) *Self Efficacy: The Exercise of Control.* W H Freeman, New York, NY.

Bhat, P.P., Rajashekar, B. & Kamath, U. (2007) Perspectives on self-directed learning – the importance of attitudes and skills. *Bioscience Education e Journal.*

Available at:http://www.bioscience.heacademy.ac.uk/journal/vol10/beej-10-c3.htm. Accessed on 27th February 2008.

Blackboard Inc. (1997) *Blackboard Academic Suite*. United States Patent No 6,988,138. Blackboard Inc., Washington, D.C.

Biggs, J. (2003) *Teaching for Quality Learning at University: What the Student Does*, 2nd edn. Open University Press, Berkshire.

Bonello, M. (2001) Fieldwork within the context of higher education: a literature review. *British Journal of Occupational Therapy*. **64** (2), 93–99.

Brookfield, S.D. (1986) *Understanding and Facilitating Adult Learning*. Open University Press, Buckingham.

Burns, R. (1995) *The Adult Learner at Work*. Business and Professional Publishing, Sydney.

Childs, P. (2005) Autonomy and the Ability to Learn. Paper presented at the 7th Annual Conference of The Learning in Law Initiative. Available at: http://www.ukcle.ac.uk/interact/lili/2005/contributions/childs.html. Accessed on 20th April 2009.

Clouston, T.J. (2005) Facilitating tutorials in problem based learning: a student's perspective. In: *Enhancing Teaching in Higher Education - New Approaches to Improving Student Learning* (eds P. Hartley, A. Woods & M, Pill), pp. 54–64. Routledge, London.

Clouston, T.J. (2007) Exploring methods of analysing talk in problem-based learning tutorials. *Journal of Further and Higher Education*. **31** (2), 183–193.

Clouston, T.J. and Whitcombe, S.W. (2005) An emerging model for problem-based learning. *Journal of Further and Higher Education*. **29** (3), 265–275.

Dolmans, D.H.J.M., De Grave, W., Wolfhagen, I.H.A.P. & van der Vleuten, C.P.M. (2005) Problem based learning: future challenges for educational practice and research. *Current perspectives*. **39**, 732–741.

Entwistle, N. (1998) *Styles of learning and teaching: an integrated outline of educational psychology for students, teachers and lecturers*. David Fulton Publishers, London.

Fazey, M.A., Fazey, J.A. (2001) The potential for autonomy in learning: perceptions of competence, motivation and locus of control in first-year undergraduate students. *Studies in Higher Education*. **26** (3), 345–361.

Fischer, G. (2000) Lifelong learning – more than training. *Journal of Interactive Learning Research*. Available at: http://www.questia.com/googleScholar.qst;jsessionid=H5SSGZPpDf4tvYgP83Xfy2rf. Accessed on 18th February 2008.

Gibbs, G. (1992) *Improving the Quality of Student Learning*. Technical and Educational services, Bristol.

Hall, E. & Moseley, D. (2005) Is there a role for learning styles in personalised education and training? *International Journal of Lifelong Education*. **24** (3), 243–255.

Harter, S. (1990) Causes, correlates and the functional role of global self worth: a life span perspective. In: *Competence Considered* (eds R.J. Sternberg & J. Kolligian), pp. 67–97. Vail-Ballou, New York, NY.

Ibrahim, M., Ogston, S., Crombie, I., Alhasso, D. & Mukhopadyay, S. (2006) Greater knowledge gain with structured than student-directed learning in child health: cluster randomized trial. *Medical Teacher*. **28** (3), 239–243.

Jamrozik, K. (1996) Clinical epidemiology: an experiment in student–directed learning in Western Australia. *Medical Education*. **30** (4), 266–271.

Jasper, M. (1995) The portfolio workbook as a strategy for student-centred learning. *Nurse Education Today.* **15** (6), 446–451.

Jette, D.U., Bertoni, A., Coots, R., Johnson, H., McLaughlin, C. & Weisbach, C. (2007) Clinical instructors' perceptions of behaviors that comprise entry-level clinical performance in physical therapist students: a qualitative study. *Physical Therapy.* **87** (7), 883–843. Available at: http://www.physicaltherapyonline.net/cgi/content/abstract/87/7/833. Accessed 26th February 2008.

Knowles, M.S. (1975) *Self-Directed Learning: A Guide for Learners and Teachers.* Cambridge The Adult Education Company, New York, NY.

Long, H.B. (2000) Understanding self-direction in learning. In: *Practice and Theory in Self-Directed Learning* (eds Long H.B. and Associates), pp. 11–24. Motorola University Press, IL.

Long, H.B. (2005) Skills for Self Directed Learning. Available at: http://faculty-staff.ou.edu/L/Huey.B.Long-1/Articles/sd/selfdirected.html. Accessed on 29th February 2008.

Mazhindu, G.N. (1990) Contract learning reconsidered: a critical examination of implications for application in nurse education. *Journal of Advanced Nursing.* **15**, 101–109.

Nolan, J. & Nolan, M. (1997) Education: self-directed and student-centred learning in nurse education. *British Journal of Nursing.* **6** (1), 51–55.

Parnell, R. (2001) It's Good to Talk: Managing Disjunction Through Peer Discussion. Available at: http://cebe.cf.ac.uk/aee/pdfs/parnellr.pdf. Accessed on 26th February 2008.

Payne, E. & Whittaker, L. (2000) *Developing Essential Study Skills.* Prentice Hall, New York, NY.

Penland, P.R. (1977) *Self-Planned Learning in America.* Book Centre, Graduate School of Library and Information Study, University of Pittsburgh, Pittsburgh, PA.

Quality Assurance Agency (2001) *Code of Practice for the Assurance of Academic Quality of Standards in Higher Education: Placement Learning.* QAA, Gloucester.

Ramsden, P. (1992) *Learning to Teach in Higher Education.* Routledge, London.

Rogers, J. (2001) *Adults Learning,* 4th edn. Open University Press, Maidenhead.

Schmidt, H.G. (2000) Assumptions underlying self-directed learning may be false. *Medical Education.* **34**, 243–245. Available at: http://www.blackwell-synergy.com/toc/med/34/4. Accessed on 29th February 2008.

Stephenson, J. & Laycock, M. (1993) Learning contracts: scope and rationale. In: *Using Learning Contracts in Higher Education* (eds J. Stephenson & M. Laycock), pp. 17–25. Kogan Page Ltd, London.

Whitcombe, S.W. (2001) Using learning contracts in fieldwork education: the views of occupational therapy students and those responsible for their supervision. *British Journal of Occupational Therapy.* **64** (11), 553–558.

Part 4

Final Thoughts

16: Interweaving the strands of thinking in problem-based learning

Teena J. Clouston

Introduction

I conclude this book by pulling together the previous chapters and inter-weaving that with my own research. I shall suggest that problem-based learning (PBL) is socially, individually and institutionally constructed and, consequently, is a co-produced phenomenon. Jasanoff (2006, p. 4) argues that co-production provides a framework for thinking about the interconnectedness between 'the macro and the micro, between emergence and stabilisation and between knowledge and practice'. Using the sociologist Pierre Bourdieu's notion of capital, habitus and field to describe this integrated relationship, I draw together the multiple strands of thinking inherent in this book to conceptualise and frame the themes of PBL into a relational form.

Problem-based learning as a relational phenomenon

As we have progressed through the book, the authors' interests and ideas about PBL have been expressed at a variety of levels. Some have focused on the agents, that is, the individual actors' viewpoints and experiences of PBL. Others have described the organisational curricula, its structure and determinants, and how that influences the process and outcomes of PBL. Further, some contributors have touched on the wider social context of learning in the United Kingdom. This latter perspective has particular relevance for curricula in health and social care because that field of learning is directed by political and professional standards that have to be evidenced and achieved in all learning environments, irrespective of the tools of delivery. In simple terms, this means that whether a traditional or a PBL approach, whether in university or in practice placement, specific frames and measurable standards have to be achieved and evidenced in the curricula.

Finally, some contributors have contextualised the ontological development of PBL, its history and roots through to potential futures. In
Chapter 2, Matheson and Haas offer an overview and historical context
of PBL. They trace the roots of PBL in biomedical learning environments
and note that this particular speciality initially promoted an analytical,
problem-based view of learning because it mirrored and enhanced the
skills needed for practice in health and social care fields. Consequently,
from its inception, PBL has had a strong affinity with developing
professional knowledge and skills, then applying that in the practice
situation. Most contributors in the book move on from this to focus
their attentions on the present opportunities, dilemmas or challenges in
PBL from a variety of perspectives. In its future contexts, Machon and
Roberts' notions of appreciative and paradoxical inquiry (Chapter 12),
challenge the taken-for-granted thinking in PBL as a problem-focused
approach, and suggest that this is actually an inherent weakness of the
PBL process, making participants search for problems and solutions
rather than building on existing strengths and the possibilities of what
works well. Whitcombe and Clouston (Chapter 9) introduce a new
model for reflexivity in PBL, and Riley and Whitcombe (Chapter 11)
suggest PBL as a proponent of social capital, a means to enrich social
connections and networks.

I am now going to briefly consider the themes within the book using
Bourdieu's relational notion of field, capital and habitus (Maton, 2005;
Swartz, 2008). I will consider the organisational settings, in Bourdieu's
term *field*, and the wider social and political frames influencing those
fields and their social actors. Using Bourdieu's analogy of a game
taking place in the field, I describe how the individual's dispositions,
in Bourdieu's terms their habitus, can effect their experience of PBL
(Bourdieu & Wacquant, 2007).

For Bourdieu, the rules of the game, in any field, were related to the
forms of capital (or power) valued in that specific field. These rules were
'a set of objective, historical relations between positions and anchored
in certain forms of power' (or capital), (Bourdieu & Wacquant, 2007,
p. 16). Bourdieu argued that players in the field were given positions
dependant on the type of capital they held. Consequently, a player's
worth was attributed in terms of how their capital was valued. Finally,
an individual's dispositions (or habitus) could only be understood in
terms of the field (or the social space) in which they were situated at
any one time. In this way, capital, habitus and field were all interrelated
and worked together to co-produce the everyday lived experiences for
individuals within any social space. When individuals move into a
different field, for example a PBL educational environment, they need
to adapt to the rules of that game. In simple terms, players have to
accommodate or achieve congruence between their own value systems

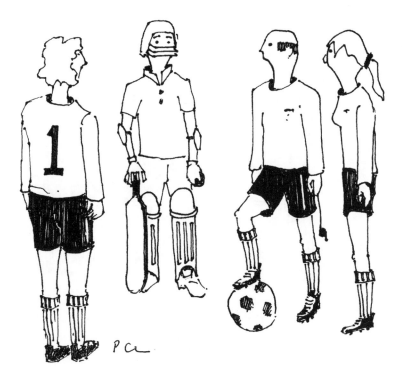

Figure 16.1 'Someone get me out of here!'.

and experiences and that of the field and its players in order to feel comfortable in that new setting. If they do not, they will always feel like they do not quite fit in (Figure 16.1).

The playing fields

Several contributors in the book have considered how PBL can enhance and develop skills within professional and educational fields as the learning experience grows. Seymour (Chapter 6) considers the use of small group work in PBL and how that can be both challenging and developmental in terms of working in teams. For me, this duality in opportunities is an important consideration in the use of PBL as a tool for learning for both students and staff alike because, as Seymour maintains, working in groups is a skilled activity. To work in this way is, of course, one of the most basic premises of effective PBL. Yet, paradoxically for participants in the process, it is possibly the most challenging aspect, because it requires the acceptance of a responsibility to work in a cooperative way (Clouston, 2007).

Talia, a student respondent in my own research (pseudonyms are used throughout), described how those who do not take this on board

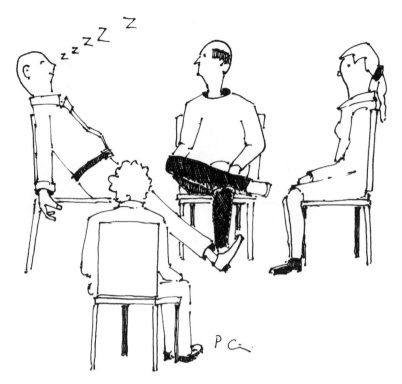

Figure 16.2 'OK ... who's done Jake's work this week?'.

could influence the whole group experience for other members. In particular, she described her concerns over the perceived inequalities in the sharing of workloads and its impact on her learning process (Figure 16.2):

> I don't like the group work. I know you say that theoretically it prepares us for working in health and social care but some people just don't work; they shirk. I mean X now, he never produces work and X [tutor] doesn't say anything. Honestly it's absolutely infuriating. I end up doing loads more work as does the rest of the group to carry the responsibility of the work that has to be done. I'm tired of it to be honest ... and it's not fair. When are we going to be marked on group work and when is that going to get me to pass this course?

Talia highlights how working in groups changes the stance of learning from an individual one to a shared one, from self-interest to utilitarianism.

She also questions how individual performance is validated and measured. It is not enough, she suggests, to just do it well; rather it should be evaluated and used as a tool of formal assessment. I feel this is a valuable point, but also suggest that it leads onto several interrelated questions. For example, what is the purpose of using small groups and what is the expected outcome? How should lack of participation be addressed and what group norms can be developed to tackle just such a problem? What is the role of the tutor in this situation and should they intervene? These issues have to be addressed and clearly delineated within the philosophical approach taken in any PBL curricula. In Bourdieu's terms, the rules of the game have to be known and understood for the game to be successful (Bourdieu & Wacquant, 2007). Without the development of these fundamentals in place, consistency in approach will be lacking and group norms will not be successfully established across the educational field. Westcott *et al.*'s chapter (Chapter 4) offers some examples of how this can influence the PBL curricula and process.

For students in health and social care, the assimilation of rules is complicated further by the roles and team-working processes adopted within the practice environment. This is a different field playing a different game with different rules. Whilst teamworking is promoted as a fundamental part of effective multidisciplinary and inter-organisational working by the New Labour Government in health and social care fields (Department of Health, 2000), like its educational counterpart, the effectiveness of this in practice is subject to many variables (Abbott & Meerabeau, 2005).

Perhaps, the most stringent influence is the professional and managerial hierarchy and its associated positions of power (Freidson, 2007). To explain this, let us go back to Bourdieu's idea of a field and use his analogy of people in that field playing a game. As noted earlier, he suggests that positions in the game are taken dependent on forms of capital (and consequently, power) individuals possess and how that is valued in the field, for example intellectual, knowledge and economic capital is valued in educational and health and social care fields (Bourdieu & Wacquant, 2007). As power is the basis of hierarchy, teamworking is always subject to that structure. This means that players in any field are positioned according to their forms of capital and provide a continuum of dominant and dominated (Bourdieu & Wacquant, 2007; Freidson, 2007). In this way, health and social care fields' professional demarcations and symbolic capital define positions and influence the rules of inter-professional working (Abbott, 1988; Freidson, 2007). Consequently, the effectiveness of PBL as a viable tool for enhancing inter-professional education or working, could, I suggest, be challenged by the power of valued forms of capital and its tacit nature in maintaining the status quo in the rules of the game.

This idea of power and capital is also intriguing in terms of the educational fields of PBL, because students, however self-directed, will always be considered to hold less intellectual and knowledge capital than tutors, and so will always be positioned in a subjugated position in the game.

In education, the tutor, whether in a facilitator role or not, assesses students' work, monitors progress and standards and it is they who, to a certain extent, decide whether students pass or fail the course. This maintains their position of power in the field and it is they who direct the learning experience, including how they approach facilitation in groups in PBL tutorials. In practice settings, such as health and social care fields, the qualified versus unqualified continuum will also place the student in a less powerful position in the field and will always project greater knowledge capital onto the qualified professional practitioner. Oriel, a student research participant recalled how she played the game whilst on placement so she could pass successfully:

> When I'm on placement I play the game . . . I do what the educator tells me to do because they're the boss at the end of the day and I want to . . . to get through.

For Oriel, *passing* was the focus and doing what she was *told* to do rather than applying the principles of self-directed learning and problem solving. It is of course the passing that would give Oriel the symbolic capital she needed to qualify as a practitioner. Griff, another student respondent, offered a similar scenario but described his challenges in the placement setting as focused more on the content of PBL learning rather than the process of it:

> My supervisor said I needed to recite the muscles of the lower limb and be able to explain their origins and insertions. I wanted to say that I didn't think it was relevant to get someone cooking in the kitchen and to evidence my understanding of human occupation. I didn't though because I wanted to pass the placement.

Galle and Marshman (Chapter 13) recount a similar experience of disjuncture between the PBL university field and the practice fields, saying they were required to do as they were told rather than take responsibility for their own learning and practice. This highlights the differences between fields and how the different rules in games can cause a sense of incongruence to occur for players who feel they have to set aside some of their own preferred dispositions (or habitus) to achieve success in the field.

From a more positive perspective, Stead, Morgan and Scott-Roberts (Chapter 14) suggest that PBL enables student participants to learn the skills necessary for lifelong learning and that this will enhance their skills and abilities to work in the changing environments of health and social care. Galle and Marshman (Chapter 13) provide some valuable support for this suggestion, offering a variety of positive skills they have developed, not only in their journeys to becoming qualified practitioners but also their reflective practice and professional development in their respective work fields.

Several contributors support the contention that PBL can provide a good basis of the development of reflective practice in health and social care fields. Boniface (Chapter 8) provides an excellent analysis of reflection and the difficulties associated with its measurement. Whitcombe and Clouston (Chapter 9) describe their model of reflexivity, suggesting that this can be used to review one's own skills and approaches to PBL and highlight previously unseen barriers, such as preconceptions and cognitive dissonance (see also Chapter 3, for more details). Of course the real challenge here, for both fields and players, is to be aware and open enough to question and enquire in such a way to feel they are being fully reflexive. This is not easy because, as Berger and Luckmann (1991) note, if the routines of everyday life continue without disruption, without question or focused awareness, then they are not perceived to be problematic.

This leads nicely to Machon and Roberts' work (Chapter 12), which sends out a tentative invitation to question the possibility for a new type of inquiry, a new way of thinking in PBL that changes the rational and accepted patterns and methods of working in PBL itself. At its most simple, these three chapters ask us to question how certain fields work, how we as individuals think in certain fields, why we do things in the way that we do (our dispositions) and offer us alternatives – different ways of thinking, a different lens through which to view PBL and to see oneself as an active participant in the process, either institutionally or individually. This of course is not easy because it requires a reflexive approach, that is, the ability to be adaptive, thinking and learning, an approach indicative of change and flexibility. For me I think a personal hero, Pooh Bear, perhaps captures this conundrum of reflexivity, waking up, being aware, questioning the accepted and taken-for-granted in everyday life and changing in its entirety:

> Here is Edward Bear, coming downstairs now, bump, bump bump on the back of his head behind Christopher Robin. It is as far as he knows the only way of coming downstairs but sometimes he feels there must be another way If only he could stop bumping for a moment and think of it.
>
> (Milne, 1994, p. 11)

With this thought in mind, let us now consider the individual players in PBL.

The individual players in PBL

As discussed above, viewing PBL through Bourdieu's lens offers an intriguing thought when thinking about PBL because as a particular sub-field in education, the traditional power hierarchy between lecturer and student are challenged to change: The lecturer lets go of his or her knowledge or intellectual capital as a symbol of power and position in the field and enacts a more facilitative role to enable the student to learn. Correspondingly, students are asked to accept positions of autonomy, to self-direct their learning process and develop their own skills in problem solving. If that is not enough, they are also expected to do this in a group situation and therefore, accept responsibility not

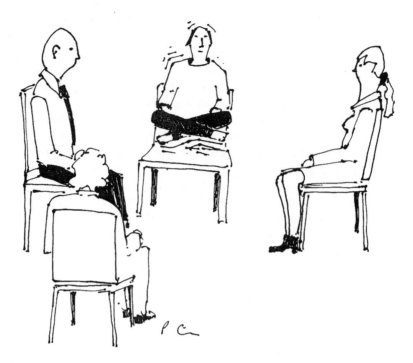

Figure 16.3 'The guru's here... We can just sit and listen.'

only for their own learning but also for other members of their group (Figure 16.3).

As many writers in this book contend, this change causes some major issues for learners and tutors who have to struggle with adjusting to those positions on the field of play. Roberts (Chapter 5) notes some of the challenges for tutors in becoming facilitators, whilst Delport and Squire describe the difficulties that can beset those specifically developing the skills of a self-directed learner (Chapter 15). Pengelly (Chapter 7) grapples admirably with thinking differently about assessments in PBL and offers some solutions about how we can assess differently to accommodate power differentials. But of course, the challenges remain, not just practically but cognitively and emotionally, and it is these two little lovelies that I wish to concentrate on here. My own research with students and tutors can give some particular examples of both of these phenomena.

Sasha, a tutor, described how he found the transition to facilitation from traditional teaching as challenging. In Bourdieu's terms, Sasha did not want to let go of his position (and power) gained through his intellectual and knowledge capital (Bourdieu & Wacquant, 2007):

> I don't know why we can't give lectures. It seems a waste of time to me to go through all the heartache of a tutorial when you can give them [students] the information. Its pressured enough isn't it. I mean I've been a therapist and I have the experience, so why can't I just share what I know?

Of course, there are many arguments to suggest that sharing knowledge and tutors being used as a resource is, in fact, an important tool in PBL, one which should be utilised by students and tutors alike (see Chapter 5, this text and Clouston, 2005 for examples). Perhaps, Sasha then, was on the right lines and merely attempting to balance the sharing and the facilitating of knowledge. It is after all, not necessarily an easy equilibrium to find. As Lilly, a student, described:

> Some tutors don't say anything at all [in tutorials]. Others take over and talk all the time. Some seem to just get the balance right and adapt it to the group's needs. That when the groups work best I think.

Tutors then, are challenged to not only adjust their own thinking but to accommodate and respond to the needs of a group. Sasha, however, went onto explain that he also felt that PBL lacked structure and consequently for him, that students were disadvantaged in their learning experience. He described a disjuncture between his work environment, the PBL field and his preferred way of teaching, which reflected his personal habitus or dispositions:

> I keep telling the others [tutors] that students need structure. They need underpinning knowledge and that's what we, as tutors, should do. We can't expect students to work independently; not without structure. They need guidance.... And that's what I want to do.

For Sasha, problem-based tutorials did not offer an appropriate tool for teaching (or learning). For Sasha as a PBL tutor, this was a point of disjuncture in his own view and that of the PBL philosophy. Delport and Whitcombe (Chapter 3) highlight the often subliminal challenges changing positions create for individuals as they negotiate their way across the field into different and often uncomfortable places (remember the first illustration?). Their chapter offers an excellent insight into the process of cognitive dissonance, a particular pitfall for PBL participants.

In Bourdieu's view, a state or cognitive dissonance or disjuncture could occur when the individual's habitus was incongruent with the field in which they were playing. He described habitus as, 'an open system of dispositions', which developed over time and were able to change and adapt to determinants in the field at any one time (Bourdieu & Wacquant, 2007, p. 133). For Bourdieu, difficulties could arise when the individual could not match their own unique life experiences or values to those inherent or ascribed to the forms of capital within a field. Riley and Whitcombe (Chapter 11) note that to an extent, habitus is in part a reflection of the values we assume and acculturate as a result of living in our social environment, in Bourdieu's terms, our cultural capital (Bourdieu & Wacquant, 2007). As Delport and Whitcombe have argued, our past experiences of learning and how we experience the PBL process can influence our readiness to work in this way. This means it can be difficult to change because the taken-for-granted patterns of behaviour, the how things are done or have been done in everyday experience and life can challenge unconsciously how the PBL process is approached. To recall Pooh's words, it is not enough to be aware that something is not quite right, then complaining about it and carrying on. It is about becoming fully aware of it, coming up with solutions or options and trying out different ways of doing things until you find one that works for you and your fellow player, because in PBL, you should not do it on your own.

Conclusion

To conclude then, if viewed from Bourdieu's perspective, the PBL process is a conglomerate of three interrelated forces: the rules of the game in the field or setting, the forms of capital that symbolise power, position and success therein and the dispositions (or habitus) of the individual as he or she plays out his or her role in their respective fields (Emirbayer, 1997; Swartz, 2008). Goffman (1974) argues that the encounters and routines in everyday life are integral to how we frame and experience everyday life. In particular, he suggests we do this in formulaic ways. Thus, the learning environment and the expected patterns that occur within are pre-empted by experience and expectations. To a certain extent, PBL challenges this because it is a non-traditional encounter in terms of the specific, socially constructed context of the learning environment. It confronts the normative, the expected or taken-for-granted ways of 'being' in the learning environment and this can mean that the roles and expectations, the enacted behaviour expected of actors in the setting is not the usual or the taken for granted (Clouston, 2007). Consequently, people might feel they do not quite 'fit' (see Figure 16.1). Yet, as Bourdieu and Riley and Matheson (Chapter 10) contend, 'we are in the world as creative and active beings' (Bourdieu & Wacquant, 2007, p. 122). This means we not only have differences in how we play the game because we have variety in life experiences allowing for unique responses in some situations (Adams, 2006), but also that we can change and experience or view things differently. As Richardson (2000, p. 934) notes, 'what we see depends upon our angle of repose'. Perhaps then, if we change our position and ways of doing and seeing things just a little more often, we would not, unlike Pooh, keep coming downstairs on the back of our heads. After all, there has to be an easier way, if only we took the time to think about it. Time is a fascinating phenomenon, which unfortunately, is not something I can discuss here; but I would suggest that if something is important enough, then the time could be found to think and act on it if you do not ignore it. To finish in the style we begun this book, I would like to end with a favourite poem by William Henry Davies (1871–1940) because it describes the problem of taking time to think about things in terms of the natural world about us. Whilst PBL lacks that importance, the poem does suggest that a little self-awareness and a lot of thought can go a long way to making life a little easier and more satisfying. Applying those principles to PBL or, indeed, any other life situation is certainly a lesson I am happy to learn.

> What is this life if full of care
> We have no time to stand and stare?
> No time to stand beneath the boughs
> And stare as long as sheep, or cows.
> No time to see, when woods we pass,
> Where squirrels hide their nuts in grass.
> No time to see, in broad daylight,
> Streams full of stars, like skies at night.
> No time to turn at Beauty's glance,
> And watch her feet, how they can dance.
> No time to wait till her mouth can
> Enrich that smile her eyes began.
> A poor life this, if full of care,
> We have no time to stand and stare.
> *Leisure* by William Henry Davies (1871–1940) (BBC Books, 1996, p. 14)

Acknowledgement

The illustrations in this chapter have been kindly supplied by Peter Cronin (Artist, www.petercronin.org). The poem *Leisure* by William Henry Davies has been reproduced by permission of Kieron Griffin as Trustee for the Mrs H.M. Davies Will Trust.

References

Abbott, A. (1988) *The System of Professions; An Essay on the Division of Expert Labour*. University of Chicago Press, Chicago, IL.

Abbott, P. & Meerabeau, L. (2005) Professionals, professionalization and the caring professions. In: *The Sociology of the Caring Professions* (eds P. Abbott & L. Meerabeau), 2nd edn. pp. 1–19. UCL Press, London.

Adams, M. (2006) Hybridizing habitus and reflexivity: toward an understanding of contemporary identity. *Sociology*. **40** (3, 5), 11–528.

BBC Books (1996) *The Nation's Favourite Poems*. BBC Worldwide Publishing, London.

Berger, P.L. & Luckmann, T. (1991) *The Social Construction of Reality: A Treatise in the Sociology of Knowledge*. Penguin, London.

Bourdieu, P. & Wacquant, L. (2007) *An Invitation to Reflexive Sociology*. Polity, Cambridge.

Clouston, T.J. (2005) Facilitating tutorials in problem-based learning: students' perspectives. In: *Enhancing Teaching in Higher Education* (eds P. Hartley, A. Woods & M. Pill), pp. 48–58. Routledge, Oxon.

Clouston, T.J. (2007) Exploring methods of analysing talk in problem-based learning tutorials. *Journal of Further and Higher Education*. **31** (2), 183–193.

Department of Health (2000) *NHS Plan: A Plan for the Future, a Plan for Reform*. Department of Health, London.

Emirbayer, M. (1997) Manifesto for a relational sociology. *American Journal of Sociology*. **103** (2), 281–317.

Freidson, E. (2007) *Professional Dominance: The Social Structure of Medical Care*. Aldine Transaction, New York, NY.

Goffman, E. (1974) *Frame Analysis: An Essay on the Organisation of Experience*. Harper Row, New York, NY.

Jasanoff, S. (2006) The idiom of co-production. In: *States of Knowledge: The Co-production of Science and the Social Order* (ed S. Jasanoff), pp. 1–12. Routledge, London.

Maton, K. (2005) A question of autonomy: Bourdieu's field approach and higher education policy. *Journal of Educaton Policy*. **20** (6), 687–704.

Milne, A.A. (1994) *Winnie-the-Pooh*. Metheun, London.

Richardson, L. (2000) Writing: a method of inquiry. In: *Handbook of Qualitative Research* (eds N.K. Denzin & Y.S. Lincoln), 2nd edn. pp. 923–948. Sage, Thousand Oaks, CA.

Swartz, D.L. (2008) Bringing Bourdieu's master concepts into organizational analysis. *Theory and Society*. **37**, 45–52.

Index

Note: Page numbers in *italics* refer to figures, those in **bold** refer to tables.